BIOMEDICAL WASTE DISPOSAL

Disclaimer

BIOMEDICAL WASTE DISPOSAL

Anantpreet Singh BDS MDS
Certificate Course in Healthcare Waste Management (IGNOU)
Lecturer, Guru Gobind Singh Medical College and Hospital
Faridkot, Punjab, India
(A Constituent College of Baba Farid University of Health Sciences, Faridkot, Punjab, India)

Sukhjit Kaur BDS PDES
Postgraduate Diploma in Clinical Research
ICRI, New Delhi, India
Demonstrator, Punjab Government Dental College and Hospital, Amritsar, Punjab, India

Foreword

SS Gill

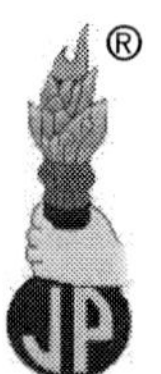

JAYPEE BROTHERS MEDICAL PUBLISHERS (P) LTD

New Delhi • Panama City • London

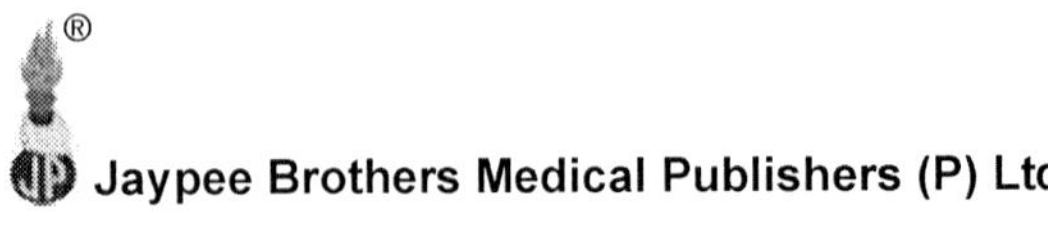

Headquarter

Jaypee Brothers Medical Publishers (P) Ltd
4838/24, Ansari Road, Daryaganj
New Delhi 110 002, India
Phone: +91-11-43574357
Fax: +91-11-43574314
Email: jaypee@jaypeebrothers.com

Overseas Offices

J.P. Medical Ltd.
83 Victoria Street, London
SW1H 0HW (UK)
Phone: +44-2031708910
Fax: +02-03-0086180
Email: info@jpmedpub.com

Jaypee-Highlights Medical Publishers Inc.
City of Knowledge, Bld. 237, Clayton
Panama City, Panama
Phone: 507-317-0160
Fax: +50-73-010499
Email: cservice@jphmedical.com

Website: www.jaypeebrothers.com
Website: www.jaypeedigital.com

Inquiries for bulk sales may be solicited at: jaypee@jaypeebrothers.com

Biomedical Waste Disposal

First Edition: **2012,** Reprint: 2025

ISBN 978-93-5025-554-4

Printed in India

Dedicated to

Our respected parents who have enabled us
to realize our dreams!

Foreword

The evolution of a separate category of medical waste within the municipal waste stream dates back to the late 1970s. The final rules were notified on 20th July, 1998 called the "Biomedical Waste (Management and Handling) Rules, 1998" followed by amendments thereto. The entire country now comes under the umbrella for implementation of the rules covering all the health-care institutions, cities, towns and villages nationally. The rules apply to all persons who generate, collect, receive, transport, treat, dispose, store, or handle biomedical waste in any form. It is the duty of the occupier, where required to set-up requisite biomedical waste treatment facilities like incinerator, autoclave, microwave for treatment of waste, or ensure requisite treatment of waste at a common waste treatment facility. However, lack of awareness among the healthcare workers in particular and public in general is posing a threat to the human beings and creating a problem in the way of implementation of these rules. They need thorough knowledge of guiding principles and their application with the accepted standards. The highest standards of safety for employees, patients and general public are required to be maintained at all the time. And, on the other hand, maintaining the detailed record of biomedical waste is a very important part of the system and is a statutory requirement.

To address the above cause, there was a long felt need of a suitable book. A literary work in the form of a book *Biomedical Waste Disposal* written by Dr Anantpreet Singh and Dr Sukhjit Kaur is a set of compilation and collection of numerous publications on the subject and provides complete information and inputs on biomedical waste disposal in all respects in an interesting, simple and easy language.

While congratulating authors for their remarkable contribution in the field of health sciences, I do hope, the book will be very useful to the entire medical fraternity.

Prof. Dr SS Gill
Vice Chancellor
Baba Farid University of Health Sciences
Faridkot, Punjab, India

Preface

Every sector has its own professional and social responsibilities. Likewise, healthcare sector too needs to be socially responsible. Apart from curing the diseases, healthcare establishments should also prevent spread of diseases. One of the main methods of disease prevention is effective biomedical waste management. To accomplish this goal, the personnel involved in such procedures should be adequately trained. The government also should frame certain rules and regulations, and the healthcare centers which do not comply with these legislations must be dealt as per law. Though with Indian Government has issued adequate guidelines in Biomedical Waste (Management and Handling) Rules, 1998 and subsequent amendments, till date, effective biomedical waste management is a distant goal when viewed throughout the country. This is partly because of lack of will at administrative level and largely because of lack of knowledge and awareness. In an endeavor to address the latter cause, a few NGOs are already working. We have also tried our best to contribute towards this social cause, by explaining every aspect of biomedical waste management.

The book is written to raise the level of awareness amongst practitioners of modern system of medicine, dental sciences, Ayurvedic and homeopathy system, nursing and other allied streams of healthcare, paramedical workers, students and general public, so as to improve the quality of environment. This will also be useful to people concerned with upkeep of environment and nature-lovers. In order to better clarify the matter in the book, a number of photographs, line diagrams and tables are added wherever required. However, various examples and figures in the book are used for the above-mentioned purpose only and do not endorse any particular brand or company. The compilation of the book involves indefinite revisions and improvement so this attempt of us is by no means to be considered a completed book. Suggestions from the readers are welcome and will be given due consideration in the subsequent editions of the book.

Anantpreet Singh
Sukhjit Kaur

Acknowledgments

We bow with reverence and all humility to thank the Almighty for His countless gracious blessings showered upon us. One of those blessings being our parents and families who have been instrumental in whatever we have achieved today.

A special debt of gratitude is owed to Dr Shivinder Singh Gill, the worthy Vice Chancellor of Baba Farid University of Health Sciences (BFUHS), Faridkot for writing foreword for this book. He always encourages his staff to excel in the field of healthcare.

The first author thanks his esteemed and revered teacher Dr Sumeet Sandhu, MDS, Professor and Head, Department of Oral and Maxillofacial Surgery, Sri Guru Ram Das Institute of Dental Sciences and Research, Amritsar, Punjab, India. He thanks her for her invaluable guidance, ever encouraging assistance, understanding nature and insight into research.

We are highly indebted to Dr Zora Singh, PhD, Department of Anatomy, (Ex-Registrar, BFUHS, Faridkot), presently working as Professor and Head, Department of Anatomy, GGS Medical College and Hospital, Faridkot for his constructive suggestions, inspiration and valuable guidance which helped us immeasurably in completing this project.

We owe thanks to Dr Vimal K Sikri, Principal, Punjab Government Dental College and Hospital, Amritsar and Dr SPS Sooch, MDS, Department of Oral and Maxillofacial Surgery, presently working as Associate Professor and Head, Department of Oral Medicine and Radiology at Punjab Government Dental College and Hospital, Amritsar for providing guidance at every step. Dr Rajeev Minhas, PhD, Library Incharge, BFUHS, Faridkot and his staff, for editing the book and providing timely suggestions.

We thank and appreciate Dr Jasbir Kaur, MDS, Associate Professor and Head, Department of Dentistry, GGS Medical College and Hospital Faridkot, for her able guidance and friendly approach at workplace.

We must acknowledge the helping hands of Dr Samir Kumar, MD, Assistant Professor, Department of Dermatology, GGS Medical College and Hospital, Faridkot, Punjab, India, for always providing constructive criticism throughout this project.

Dr Pardeep Goyal, MDS, Consultant, Oral and Maxillofacial Surgeon, SGL Superspeciality Hospital, Jalandhar, Punjab, India, deserves special thanks as he always lends a helping hand whenever we need any support. Also, he has been our main motivator to take up this project.

We would also commend with appreciation the services of Mr Sadanand (Pioneer Computers, Amritsar) for their speed and accuracy in typing; and Mr Sarbjeet Singh, MSc, Computer Sciences, Programmer, BFUHS, Faridkot for styling the book.

The cooperation from different authors, writers and agencies [WHO, CDC, CPCB and its state bodies (especially Punjab Pollution Control Board), Environment Canada, Ontario Dental Association, Toxics Link] is highly appreciated and duly acknowledged. The citations throughout the book are also duly acknowledged.

Last but not least, we feel privileged to thank our publishers M/s Jaypee Brothers Medical Publishers (P) Ltd, New Delhi, India and their staff especially Mr Tarun Duneja, (Director–Publishing) for abundant cooperation and skillful approach to shape this manuscript into a beautiful transcript.

Contents

PLATE 1

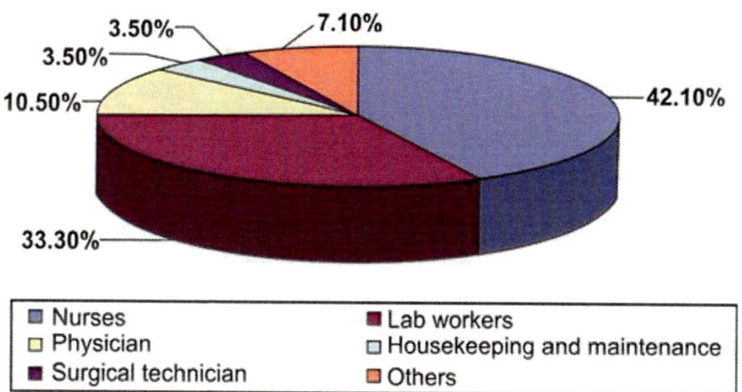

Fig. 5.1: Pie chart showing statistics about healthcare workers who acquired HIV/ AIDS at work during 1981–2002

Source: *Worker Chartbook 2004 NIOSH Publication No. 2004-146*

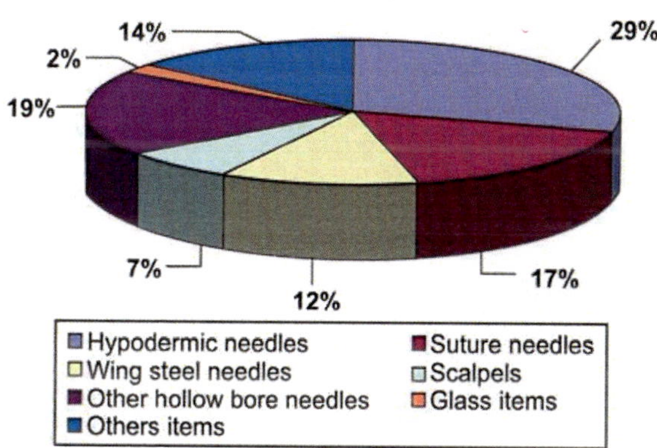

Fig. 5.2: Statistics about medical devices associated with percutaneous injuries during 1995–2000

Source: *Worker Health Chartbook 2004 NIOSH Publication No. 2004-146*

PLATE 2

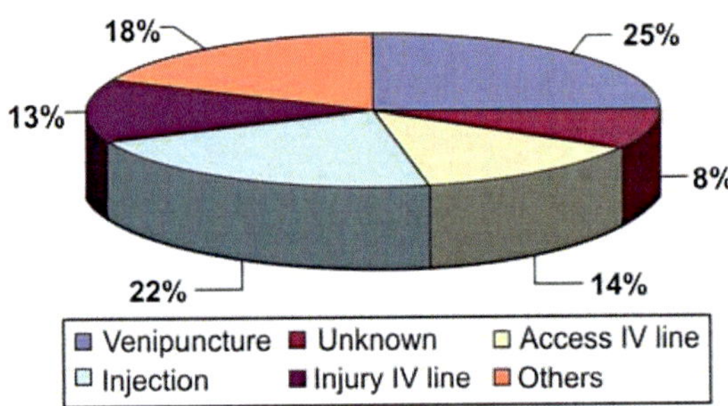

Fig. 5.3: Statistics about medical procedures involving hollow-bore needles associated with percutaneous injuries during 1995–2000

Source: *Worker Health Chartbook 2004 NIOSH Publication No. 2004-146*

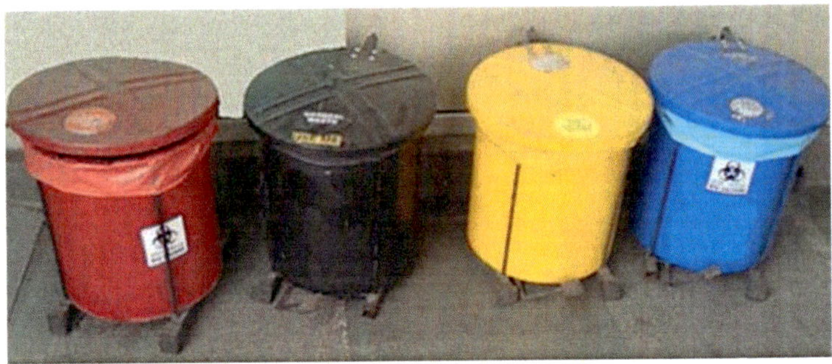

Fig. 8.1: Color-coded containers

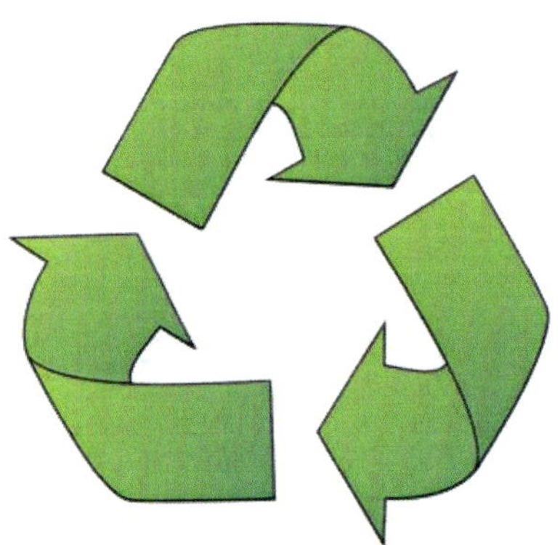

Fig. 8.5: Recyclable waste

CHAPTER 1

Introduction

To cater to the needs of the expanding population, the last century witnessed rapid mushrooming of healthcare establishments in both government and in private sector.[19,30] With the advent, acceptance and increasing demand of "disposable items", the present hospitals generate of healthcare wastes in substantial amount.[19] The absence of proper waste management, lack of awareness about the associated health hazards, human resources, insufficient financial and poor control of waste disposal are the main contentious issues connected with healthcare wastes.[63,100]

Thus inadequate, inappropriate and improper waste management leads to foul odor, environmental pollution, multiplication of disease carrying organisms like insects, rodents and worms and hence the transmission of diseases like typhoid, cholera, hepatitis A, B, C and AIDS through contact with infected waste and in particular through accidental injuries from used sharps.[19] Owing to unsafe healthcare practices, half a million people all over the world die every year due to infections like hepatitis B, and C, HIV and hepatocellular carcinoma.[7,97] Apart from these health risks, inappropriate management of healthcare wastes also has a negative impact on environment by adding toxic pollutants to water, air and soil. This environmental pollution can potentially damage our flora, fauna and the ecosystem.[19]

Not only are the healthcare workers at risk of acquiring infection through improper handling hospital wastes, but also general public is exposed to avoidable risks. The risk to the public increases many folds as disposable items are picked up by rag pickers in India and recirculated into the market without any sterilization.[19,96] In an assessment report of WHO of 2002, covering 22 developing countries, it is stated that 18 to 64 percent of healthcare facilities do not use proper waste disposal methods ranges.[99]

According to World Health Organization, 85 percent of hospital wastes are nonhazardous, whereas 15 percent are hazardous wastes, subcategorized as 10 percent being infectious and 5 percent are non-infectious.[70] Developed countries generate approximately 1 to 5 kg of hospital waste/bed/day, whereas developing countries add 1 to 2 kg/bed/day.[69] In developed countries like US and Canada, annual waste production in over 1 million hospital beds is about 2 tonnes per hospital bed, or about 2,000,000 tonnes in total.[71]

In India, the estimated figure is 2.0 kg/bed/day and out of this, 10 to 15 percent is found to biomedical waste.[19] India, the highest generator of biomedical waste in the world, contributes 0.33 million tonnes per year.[77]

Biomedical waste means any waste, which is generated during the diagnosis, treatment or immunization of human beings or animals or in research activities pertaining thereto or in the production or testing of biologicals, and including categories listed in Schedule I.[83]

The biomedical waste and their appropriate disposal has come up as a challenge and hence have become an issue of increasing concern. Public has become more aware and conscious about the production of hazardous wastes and subsequent methods employed for its disposal. This has prompted hospital administration experts to find new ways of scientific, safe and cost-effective management of the biomedical waste.[19] To address these public concerns and acting upon the directives of honorable Supreme Court of India, Biomedical Waste (Management and Handling) or BMW Rules, 1998 were drafted in exercise of powers conferred by Section 6, 8 and 25 of the Environment (Protection) Act, 1986 that was published in The Gazette of India Extraordinary, Part-II, Section 3-Subsection (ii) New Delhi, July 27, 1998.[6]

As per the Biomedical Waste (Management and Handling) rules, 1998, it is the responsibility of every occupier of an institution generating biomedical waste (which includes hospitals, nursing homes, clinics, dispensaries, veterinary institutions, animal houses, pathological laboratories, blood banks, etc.), that all necessary steps are taken for handling such wastes without any adverse effect to human health and environment.[56] The healthcare establishments would also follow strict segregation, packaging, labeling and disposal as per the BMW Rules, 1998.[79]

In India particularly many institutions lack appropriate systems because of nonavailability of appropriate technologies, lack of professional training and adequate financial resources and above all lack of commitment at each level.[63] However, many NGOs and media personnel are actively working in this field and trying to bring this issue to the fore.

CHAPTER

2 Types of Wastes

WASTE

"Waste" means any useless, unwanted or discarded substance or material, whether or not such substance or material has any other or future use and includes any substance or material that is spilled, leaked, pumped, poured, emitted, emptied or dumped onto the land or into the water or ambient air.[25]

GENERAL WASTE

General waste is nonhazardous waste such as kitchen waste, paper or wrappers, etc. It contributes 85 to 90 percent to the total healthcare waste.

This waste follows the domestic waste stream as it does not require any special treatment. However, meticulous segregation is must to keep it separate from infected or hazardous waste.[46]

BIOMEDICAL WASTE

Biomedical waste is any waste, which is generated during the diagnosis, treatment or immunization of human beings or animals or in research activities pertaining thereto or in the production or testing of biologicals, and including categories mentioned in Schedule I.[51]

It also includes the waste originating from 'minor' or 'scattered' sources, e.g. wastes produced during healthcare at home, i.e. dialysis, insulin injections, etc. Between 75 percent and 90 percent of the waste produced by any housekeeping functions and administrative functions of healthcare establishments (including waste generated during maintenance of healthcare premises) is nonrisk or general healthcare waste. This waste is comparable to domestic waste. So general healthcare wastes can be treated or disposed of in a similar, i.e. the municipal waste disposal. The remaining 10 to 25 percent of healthcare waste is regarded as hazardous and may create a variety of health risks.

Infectious Waste

Infectious waste is suspected to contain pathogenic organisms, i.e. bacteria, viruses, parasites, or fungi in sufficient concentration or quantity to cause disease in susceptible hosts. This category includes the following wastes:

- Cultures and stocks of infectious agents from clinical laboratories.
- Wastes from surgery and autopsies done on patients suffering from infectious diseases (e.g. tissues, materials or equipment that have been in contact with blood or other body fluids).
- Excreta, dressings from infected/surgical wounds, clothes heavily soiled with human blood or other body fluids, etc. from infected patients in isolation wards.
- Dialysis equipment such as tubing and filters, gowns, aprons, gloves, disposable towels and laboratory coats which have been in contact with infected patients undergoing hemodialysis.
- Infected research animals from laboratories.
- Any other instruments or materials that have been in contact with infected persons or animals.
- Cultures and stocks of highly infectious organisms, waste from autopsies, animal bodies, and other waste items inoculated, infected, or in contact with such agents are called highly infectious wastes.

Pathological Waste

Pathological waste consists of tissues, organs, body parts, human fetuses and animal carcasses, blood, and body fluids. Anatomical waste, i.e. recognizable human or animal body parts also comes under this category. Even though this category may include healthy body parts, it should be considered as a subcategory of infectious waste.

Sharps

Sharps are items that could cause cuts or puncture wounds, including needles, hypodermic needles, scalpel and other blades, knives, infusion sets, saws, broken glass, and nails. Irrespective of the associated infection potential, such items are usually considered as highly hazardous healthcare waste.

Pharmaceutical Waste

Pharmaceutical waste includes expired, unused, spilt, and contaminated pharmaceutical products, drugs, vaccines, and sera that are no longer required and require appropriate disposal. Also included are the discarded items used in the handling of pharmaceuticals, such as bottles or boxes with residues, gloves, masks, connecting tubing, and drug vials.

Genotoxic Waste

Genotoxic waste is highly hazardous and it may have mutagenic, teratogenic, or carcinogenic properties. It poses serious safety threats, both inside hospitals and after disposal. It includes certain cytostatic drugs, feces, urine, or vomit from patients treated with cytostatic drugs, chemicals, and radioactive materials. The principal substances in this category, cytotoxic or antineoplastic drugs, have the ability to kill or stop the growth of certain living cells. Due to this property, they are used in chemotherapy of cancer.

Most common genotoxic products used in healthcare

A. Classified as Carcinogenic

Chemicals

Benzene

Cytotoxic and other drugs

Azathioprine, Chlorambucil, Chlornaphazine, Cyclosporin, Cyclophosphamide, Melphalan, Semustine, Tamoxifen, Thiotepa, Treosulfan.

B. Classified as Possibly or Probably Carcinogenic

Cytotoxic and Other Drugs

Azacitidine, Bleomycin, Carmustine, Chloramphenicol, Chlorozotocin, Cisplatin, Dacarbazine, Daunorubicin, Dihydroxymethylfuratrizine, Doxorubicin, Lomustine, Methylthiouracil, Metronidazole, Mitomycin, Nafenopin, Niridazole, Oxazepam, Phenacetin, Phenobarbital, Phenytoin, Procarbazine Hydrochloride, Progesterone, Sarcolysin, Streptozocin, Trichlormethine.

Sources of Cytotoxic Wastes

- Contaminated materials generated during preparation and administration of drugs, i.e. syringes, needles, gauges, vials, packaging materials.
- Outdated drugs, excess or leftover solutions, drugs returned from the wards.
- Feces, urine and vomit from patients treated with cytostatic drugs. These excreta may contain potentially hazardous amounts of the administered cytostatic drugs or of their metabolites. These wastes should be considered genotoxic for at least 48 hours and sometimes up to 1 week after drug administration.

In specialized oncological hospitals, genotoxic waste may constitute up to 1 percent of the total healthcare wastes.

Chemical Waste

Chemical waste consists of discarded solid, liquid and gaseous chemicals, i.e. those generated from diagnostic and experimental work and from procedures like cleaning, housekeeping and disinfection. Chemical waste from healthcare may be:

a. Hazardous
b. Nonhazardous.

Waste it is considered to be hazardous if it has at least one of the following properties:

- **Toxic** *(Fig. 2.1)*;
- **Corrosive (e.g. acids of pH < 2 and bases of pH > 12)** *(Fig. 2.2)*;
- **Flammable** *(Fig. 2.3)*;

- **Reactive (explosive, water-reactive, shock-sensitive)** *(Fig. 2.4)*;
- **Genotoxic (e.g. cytostatic drugs).**

On the other hand, nonhazardous chemical waste consists of chemicals with none of the above properties, such as sugars, amino acids, and certain organic and inorganic salts. The types of hazardous chemicals used most commonly in maintenance of healthcare centers and hospitals are given below.

Formaldehyde

Formaldehyde constitutes a major part of chemical waste in hospitals. Its range of usage in hospital varies from cleaning and disinfection of equipment (e.g. surgical or hemodialysis equipment),

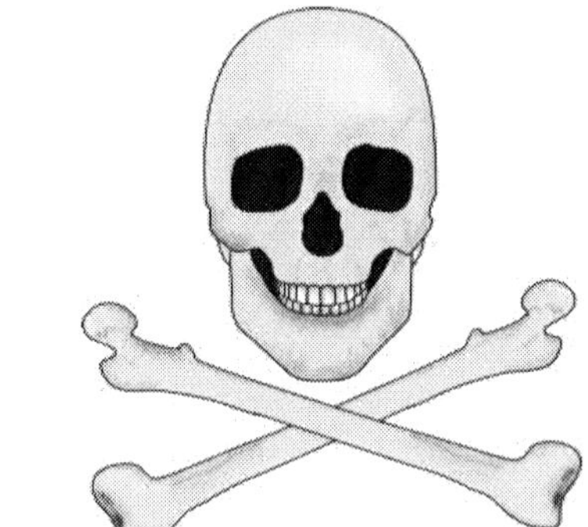

Fig. 2.1: Toxic

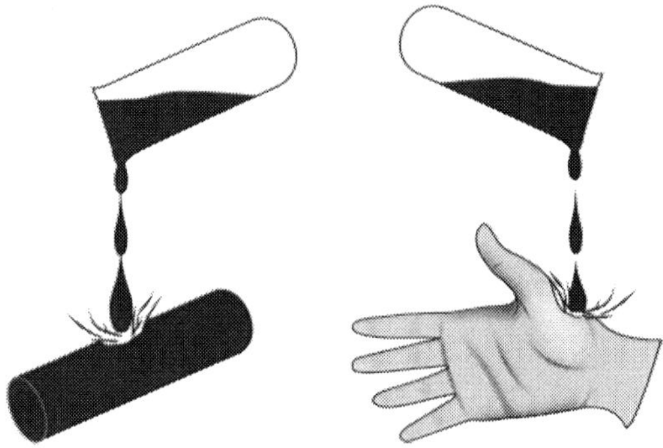

Fig. 2.2: Corrosive

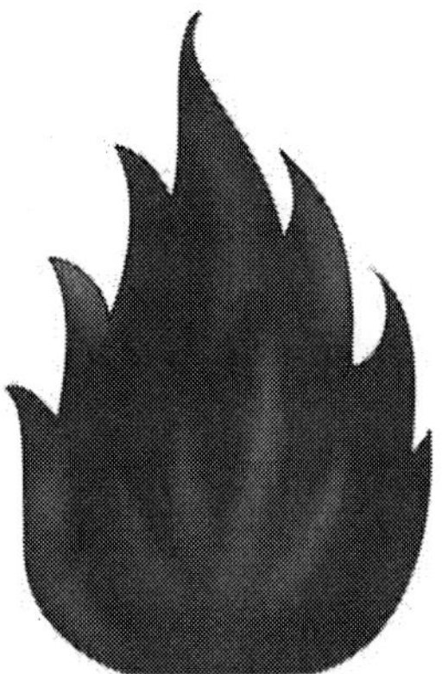

Fig. 2.3: Flammable

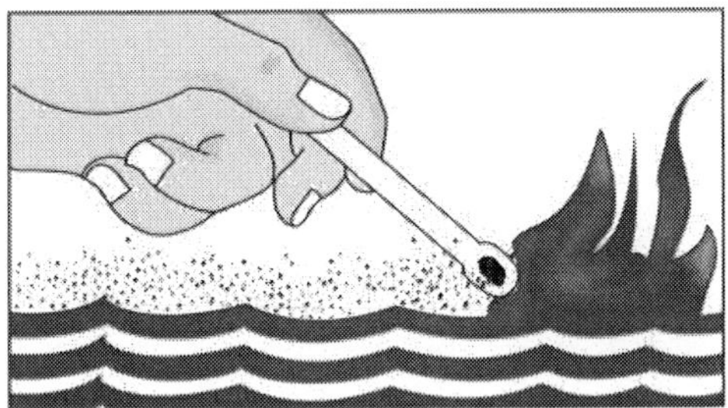

Fig. 2.4: Reactive

preservation of specimens, disinfecting liquid infectious waste, etc. to use in autopsy, pathology, dialysis, embalming and nursing units.

Solvents

Various departments of a hospital, including pathology and histology laboratories and engineering departments, generate wastes containing solvents. These solvents are halogenated compounds (e.g. methylene chloride, chloroform, trichloroethylene and refrigerants), and nonhalogenated compounds (e.g. xylene, methanol, isopropanol, acetone, toluene, acetonitrile, ethyl acetate, etc).

Photographic/Radiographic Chemicals

The fixer and developer solutions used in X-ray departments contain hazardous chemicals. The fixer usually contains hydroquinone 5 to 10 percent, potassium hydroxide 1 to 5 percent, silver <1 percent and acetic acid whereas the developer solution contains glutaraldehyde (approximately 45%) and acetic acid as hazardous chemicals.

Organic Chemicals

Waste organic chemicals generated in healthcare establishments include:

- Disinfecting and cleaning solutions: For example, phenol based chemicals are used for scrubbing floors, perchlorethylene is used in laundries and workshops.
- Oils: Vacuum-pump oils, used engine oil from vehicles, etc.
- Insecticides and rodenticides.

Inorganic Chemicals

Waste inorganic chemicals consist mainly of acids (e.g. sulfuric, hydrochloric, nitric, and chromic acids), alkalis (e.g. sodium hydroxide and ammonia solutions), oxidants (e.g. potassium permanganate and potassium dichromate) and reducing agents (e.g. sodium sulfite and sodium bisulfite).

Wastes with high content of heavy metals

Wastes with high heavy metal content (mercury, cadmium, lead, arsenic, etc.) are usually highly toxic. The sources of mercury containing wastes are spillage from broken clinical equipment and elemental mercury and scrap amalgam from dental offices. However, the volume of these wastes is decreasing with the substitution of equipment with solid-state electronic sensing instruments (e.g. thermometers, blood pressure gauges, etc.) and increased use of alternative restorative materials in dentistry. Cadmium waste enters the waste stream mainly from discarded batteries. Certain lead containing reinforced wood panels are still used for protection against X-rays and in diagnostic departments. Arsenic compounds are still used for pharmaceutical purposes. Arsenic trioxide is used treatment of for acute promyelocytic leukemia in patients who are unresponsive to, or have relapsed chemotherapy agents. Arsenic causes skin lesions and carcinomas of the bladder, kidney, liver, lung, colon, uterus, prostate, vascular, reproductive, developmental and neurological effects.

Pressurized containers

Gases used in healthcare are often stored in pressurized cylinders, cartridges, and aerosol cans. Many of these discarded containers are reusable, but aerosol cans are disposable only.

These pressurized containers may explode if incinerated or accidentally punctured. So they should be handled with extra care.

Most Commonly Used Gases in Healthcare

Anesthetic Gases

Nitrous oxide and volatile halogenated hydrocarbons (e.g. halothane, isoflurane, and enflurane) are the most commonly used anesthetic gases these days.

Applications

- In hospital operating theaters
- During childbirth in maternity hospitals
- In ambulances
- In general hospital wards during painful procedures
- In dentistry for sedation.

Ethylene Oxide

Applications

- For sterilization of surgical equipment and medical devices
- In central supply areas
- At times, in operating rooms.

Oxygen

Stored in bulk tank or cylinders, in gaseous or liquid form, or is supplied by central piping.

Application

- Inhalation supply for patients.

Compressed Air

Applications

- In laboratory work
- Inhalation therapy equipment
- Maintenance equipment
- Environmental control systems.

Radioactive waste

Radioactive waste includes solid, liquid and gaseous wastes contaminated with radionuclides from nuclear medical diagnostic and therapeutic procedures. Disposal of such waste require special techniques. Waste in the form of sealed sources may be of fairly high activity, but is only generated in low volumes from larger medical and research laboratories.

The most common radionuclides used in diagnostic nuclear medicine and the maximum activity per diagnostic test are listed in Table 2.1.

Principal Radionuclides Used in Healthcare Establishments

Sealed Sources

Sealed sources are usually contained in equipment or as needles or seeds that may be reused after sterilization for other patients.

Unsealed Sources

Unsealed sources of radioactive material used in healthcare facilities usually results in low level radioactive wastes (<1MBq), but sealed sources may produce waste of fairly high activity. Usually the radioactive healthcare waste contains radionuclides of short half lives like ^{32}P (β, 14.3 days half-life), $^{99}Tc_m$ (γ, 14.3 days half-life) ^{57}Co or (β, 271 days half-life) which lose their activity relatively quickly. However, certain therapeutic procedures require longer half-life radionuclides like ^{60}Co (β, 30 years half-life) or ^{226}Ra (β, 1600 years half-life). These are usually conditioned as pins, or seeds that may be reused after sterilization for other patients.

Table 2.1: Principal radionuclides used in healthcare establishments

Radionuclide	*Emission*	*Format*	*Half-life*	*Application*
^{3}H	β	Unsealed	12.3 years	Research
^{14}C	β	Unsealed	5730 years	Research
^{32}P	β	Unsealed	14.3 days	Diagnosis: therapy
^{51}Cr	γ	Unsealed	27,8 days	*in vitro* diagnosis
^{57}Co	β	Unsealed	271 days	*in vitro* diagnosis
^{60}Co	β	Sealed	5.3 years	Diagnosis therapy; research
^{59}Fe	β	Unsealed	45 days	*in vitro* diagnosis
^{67}Ga	γ	Unsealed	78 hours	Diagnostic imaging
^{75}Se	γ	Unsealed	119 days	Diagnostic imaging
^{85}Kr	β	Unsealed	10.7 years	Diagnostic imaging; research
^{99m}Tc	γ	Unsealed	S hours	Diagnostic imaging
^{123}I	γ	Unsealed	13.1 hours	Diagnostic uptake; therapy
^{125}I	γ	Unsealed	60 days	Diagnostic uptake; therapy
^{131}I	β	Unsealed	8 days	Therapy
^{133}Xe	β	Unsealed	5.3 days	Diagnostic imaging
^{137}Cs	β	Sealed	30 years	Therapy; research
^{192}Ir	β	Sealed (ribbons)	74 days	Therapy
^{198}Au	β	Sealed (seeds)	2.3 days	Therapy
^{222}Rd	α	Sealed (seeds)	3.8 days	Therapy
^{226}Ra	α	Sealed	1600 years	Therapy

^{3}H and ^{14}C used for research purposes account for the largest amount of radioactive healthcare waste.

Source: *Pruss A, Giroult E, Rushbrook, Safe Management of Waste from Healthcare activities (WHO).*

The radioactive waste produced by healthcare and research activities can be classified as:

- Sealed sources
- Spent radionuclide generators
- Low level solid waste, e.g. absorbent paper, swabs, glassware, syringes, vials

- Residues from shipments of radioactive material and unwanted solutions of radionuclides intended for diagnostic or therapeutic use
- Liquid immiscible with water, such as liquid scintillation-counting residues used in radioimmunoassay and contaminated pump oil
- Waste from spills and from decontamination of radioactive spills
- Excreta from patients treated or tested with unsealed radionuclides
- Low level liquid waste, e.g. from washing apparatus
- Gases and exhausts from stores and fume cupboards.[66]

CHAPTER

3 Major and Minor Sources of Biomedical Waste

In a hospital produces, every ward produces peculiar composition of waste because of difference in materials and methods of treatment of its patient's, for examples:

- *Medical wards*: Mainly infectious waste such as dressings, bandages, used hypodermic needles, intravenous sets, gloves, disposable medical items, sticking plaster, body fluids and excreta, contaminated packaging, and meal scraps.
- *Operation theaters and surgical wards*: In addition to above-mentioned wastes, mainly anatomical waste such as tissues, organs, body parts, including fetuses.
- *Immunization ward*: Hypodermic needles and syringes, residual vaccine, cotton swabs and ampoules, etc.
- *Other healthcare wards*: Mostly general waste with a small percentage of infectious waste.
- *Laboratories*: Mainly pathological and highly infectious waste, e.g. small pieces of tissue, infected animal carcasses, microbiological cultures, stocks of infectious agents, blood and other body fluids plus sharps, some radioactive and chemical waste.
- *Pharmaceutical and chemical stores*: Only small quantities of pharmaceutical and chemicals wastes, mainly packaging (containing only residues if stores are well-managed), and general waste.
- *Support units*: Only general waste.

Healthcare waste generated at various sources generally has the characteristic composition, for examples:

- *General physician's clinics*: Infectious waste and some sharps.
- *Dental clinics*: Infectious wastes, sharps, and wastes with high heavy metal content, (e.g. mercury, silver, etc.).
- *Nurse's station*: Infectious waste and many sharps.
- *Home healthcare,* e.g. dialysis, insulin injections: Mainly infectious waste and sharps.[66]

WASTE GENERATION

Reports from developed countries like USA and Canada show that approximately 1 to 5 kg of waste is generated per bed per day, whereas the figure from developing countries is 1 to 2 kg/bed/day. It is estimated to be 2.0 kg/bed/day in India.[69] A number of factors influence the quantity and quality of waste viz:

a. Type of hospital and its specialties
b. Whether proper waste management plan is implemented or not
c. Ratio of disposable/reusable items.[46]

Though not many national level studies have been conducted so far to determine quantity of hospital waste generated per bed per day, local or regional level studies in various hospitals can be used to safely presume that most hospitals generate approx. 1 to 2 kg/bed/day of waste.

In various hospitals of four major cities. In India, the quantity and type of waste generated is given below[101] (Table 3.1).

Major Sources of Healthcare Waste

Hospitals

- Healthcare teaching institutions and hospitals
- General hospitals
- District hospitals.

Table 3.1: Quantity of waste generated in various places in India

Sr. No.	City/place	Type of hospital	Quantum of waste (Kg/bed/day)	Composition %
1.	Mumbai TMH	Tertiary care cancer hospital	1.13	46% infectious
2.	New Delhi Vatavaran NIHFWO	Govt. and Pvt. hospitals Govt. teaching Hospitals	2.2 Kg	45% infectious
	AIIMS	Tertiary care (research hospitals)	1.4 to 1.6 Kg	
3.	Kolkata AIIPH	Govt., private nursing homes (large hospitals)	1.044-1.368	20-30% infectious 50-75% general
4.	Manipal KMC Manipal	Large tertiary care hospital	0.775 Kg	16.26% infectious

Source: *Yadav M. Hospital Waste: A major problem (2001)*

Other Healthcare Establishments

- Emergency medical care services
- Obstetric and maternity clinics
- Healthcare centers and dispensaries
- Outpatient clinics
- Transfusion centers
- Military medical services
- Dialysis centers
- First-aid posts and sick bays
- Long-term healthcare establishments and hospitals.

Blood banks and blood collection services
Related laboratories and research centers
Medical and autopsy centers
Animal research and testing.

Minor Sources of Healthcare Waste

Small Healthcare Establishments

- Physician's offices
- Dental clinics
- Chiropractors
- Acupuncturists.

Specialized Healthcare Establishments and Institutions with Low Waste Generation

- Psychiatric hospitals
- Convalescent nursing homes
- Disabled person's institutions.

Intravenous or Subcutaneous Intervention Activities Other than Healthcare

- Cosmetic body-piercing and tattoo parlors
- Illicit drug users.

Ambulance services
Home treatments
Funeral services.[66]

CHAPTER

4 Categories and Classification of Biomedical Wastes

Biomedical waste is extremely hazardous type of waste. If it is not managed properly, it poses serious health and environment problems.[44] Biomedical waste means any waste, which is generated during the diagnosis, treatment or immunization of human beings or animals or in research activities pertaining thereto or in the production or testing of biologicals, and including categories mentioned listed in Schedule I.[52]

OBJECTIVES OF BIOMEDICAL WASTE MANAGEMENT

Objectives of biomedical waste management are:

- Prevention of transmission of diseases from patient to patient, patient to health worker and *vice versa*
- Prevention of injury to the healthcare worker and workers in support services during handling of biomedical waste
- Prevention of exposure to the harmful effects of the genotoxic, cytotoxic, and chemical biomedical waste.[83]

Concerned over the seriousness of the issue, Ministry of Environment and Forest (MoEF) proposed the first draft rules in 1995. The rules recommended that all hospitals with more than 50 beds should have onsite incinerators. The honorable Supreme Court of India, took a similar and simultaneous decision in a public interest case in March 1996, and ordered the inclusion of alternate technologies and their standards in the BMW rules. So the second draft rules were notified in 1997. The final rules (July 1998) were called Biomedical Waste (Management and Handling) or BMW Rules 1998 in exercise of powers conferred by Section 6, 8 and 25 of the Environment (Protection) Act, 1986 that was published in The Gazette of India Extraordinary, Part-II, Section 3 Subsection (ii) New Delhi, July 27, 1998. A first amendment (March 2000) changed Schedule VI of the rules, concerning

CATEGORIES OF BIOMEDICAL WASTE (AS GIVEN IN BMW RULES, 1998)

SCHEDULE I		
Option	*Waste category*	*Treatment and disposal*
Category No. 1	**Human Anatomical Waste** (Human tissues, organs, body parts)	Incinerations@/deep burial*
Category No. 2	**Animal Waste** (Animal tissues, organs, body parts carcasses, bleeding parts, fluid, blood and experimental animals used in research, waste generated by veterinary hospitals colleges, discharge from hospitals, animal houses)	Incinerations@/deep burial*
Category No. 3	**Microbiology and Biotechnology Waste** (Wastes from laboratory cultures, stocks or specimens of micro-organisms live or attenuated vaccines, human and animal cell culture used in research and infectious agents from research and industrial laboratories, wastes from production of biologicals, toxins, dishes and devices used for transfer of cultures)	Local autoclaving/microwaving/incineration@
Category No. 4	**Waste Sharps** (Needles, syringes, scalpels, blades, glass, etc. that may cause puncture and cuts. This includes both used and unused sharps)	Disinfection (chemical treatment@01/autoclaving/microwaving and mutilation/shredding
Category No. 5	**Discarded Medicines and Cytotoxic Drugs** (Wastes comprising of outdated, contaminated and discarded medicines)	Incineration@/destruction and drugs disposal in secured landfills

Contd...

Contd...

Option	*Waste category*	*Treatment and disposal*
Category No. 6	**Solid Waste** (Items contaminated with blood, and body fluids including cotton, dressings, soiled plaster casts, lines, beddings, other material contaminated with blood)	Incineration@ autoclaving/microwaving
Category No. 7	**Solid Waste** (Wastes generated from disposable items other than the waste sharps such as tubings, catheters, intravenous sets, etc.)	Disinfection by chemical treatment@@ autoclaving/ microwaving and mutilation/ shredding##
Category No. 8	**Liquid Waste** (Waste generated from laboratory and washing, cleaning, housekeeping and disinfecting activities)	Disinfection by chemical treatment@@ and discharge into drains
Category No. 9	**Incineration Ash** (Ash from incineration of any biomedical waste)	Disposal in municipal landfill
Category No. 10	**Chemical Waste** (Chemicals used in production of biologicals, chemicals used in disinfection, as insecticides, etc.)	Chemical treatment@@ and discharge into drains for liquids and secured landfill for solids

@@ Chemicals treatment using at least 1% hypochlorite solution or any other equivalent chemical reagent. It must be ensured that chemical treatment ensures disinfection.

Mutilation/shredding must be such so as to prevent unauthorized reuse.

@ There will be no chemical pretreatment before incineration. Chlorinated plastics shall not be incinerated.

* Deep burial shall be an option available only in towns with population less than five lakhs and in rural areas.

Note: The amended version of Biomedical Waste (Management and Handling) Rules, 1998 is given in appendix.

Biomedical waste shall be segregated into containers/bags at the point of generation in accordance with schedule II prior to its storage, transportation, treatment and disposal.

having waste management facilities for treatment of waste. The second amendment to the rules (June, 2000) nominated Pollution Control Boards/Committees as Prescribed Authorities, since the work involved a lot of technical intervention like monitoring the air emission from the incinerators and the waste water effluents. Another amendment, in which guidelines for armed forces were drafted, was added in 2003.[6,100]

SCHEDULE II
COLOR CODING AND TYPE OF CONTAINER FOR DISPOSAL OF BIOMEDICAL WASTES

Color coding	*Type of container*	*Waste category*	*Treatment options as per Schedule I*
Yellow	Plastic bag	Cat.1, Cat. 2, Cat.3, Cat. 6	Incineration/deep burial
Red	Disinfected container/ plastic bag	Cat. 3, Cat. 6, Cat. 7	Autoclaving/microwaving/ chemical treatment
Blue/white translucent	Plastic bag/ puncture proof container	Cat. 4, Cat. 7	Autoclaving/microwaving/ chemical treatment and destruction/shredding
Black	Plastic bag	Cat. 5, and Cat. 9 and Cat. 10 (solid)	Disposal in secured landfill

Notes:
1. Color coding of waste categories with multiple treatment options as defined in Schedule I, shall be selected depending on treatment option chosen, which shall be as specified in Schedule I.
2. Waste collection bags for waste types needing incineration shall not be made of chlorinated plastics.
3. Categories 8 and 10 (liquid) do not require containers/bags.
4. Category 3 if disinfected locally need not to be put in containers/bags.[52]

CLASSIFICATION OF BIOMEDICAL WASTE

A number of methods have been used by various agencies for the classification of biomedical waste. These include the following:
1. **WHO Classification for developing countries**
   - General nonhazardous wastes
   - Infected wastes (not containing sharps)

- Sharps
- Chemical and pharmaceutical wastes
- Other hazardous waste—cytotoxic and radioactive.[26]

2. **Classification based on nature of waste.**

Hazardous Waste

A. *Potentially infectious waste*

Infectious waste has been mentioned under various terms, in the scientific literature, in regulation and in the guidance manuals and standards viz. infectious/infective/medical/biomedical/ contaminated/red bag/hazardous/medical infectious/regulated medical waste and regulated waste. It makes about 10 percent of the total waste and includes:

1. Potentially infected material: Such as excised tumors and organs, placenta removed during surgery, etc.
2. Potentially infected animals which are used in diagnostic and research studies.
3. Laboratory waste such as lab culture stocks of infectious agents.
4. Dressings and swabs, etc. contaminated with blood, pus and body fluids.
5. Blood and blood products.
6. Sharps including blades, needle, syringes, etc.

B. *Potentially toxic waste*

1. *Radioactive waste:* It means waste contaminated with radionuclides in the form of solid, liquid or gaseous waste. These wastes are generated during *in vitro* analysis of body fluids and tissue, therapeutic procedures and *in vitro* imaging.
2. *Chemical waste:* It includes disinfectants (sodium hypochlorite, glutaraldehyde, phenolic derivatives, iodophors and alcohol-based preparations), X-ray processing solutions, etc.
3. *Pharmaceutical waste:* It includes antibiotics, anesthetics, analgesics, sedatives, etc.

Nonhazardous Waste

It constitutes about 85 percent of the waste generated in most healthcare establishments. This includes waste comprising of food remnants, fruit peels, waste paper, packaging material, etc.[40]

CHAPTER 5

Hazards of Biomedical Waste

Ideally waste from healthcare establishments should be collected and segregated for proper treatment. Also measures should be taken to transport it to waste disposal site in a hygienic manner and treat it in a scientific manner. But in our country, only 41.2 percent of biomedical waste is handled properly. Rest of this biomedical waste is mixed with general waste. Municipalities collect this waste and dispose it off in outskirts of the cities and towns.

The biomedical waste (BMW) emits a foul smell during the rainy season and acts as potential breeding ground for flies, mosquitoes, rodents and insects. Due to these acts, diseases like hepatitis, tetanus and dengue fever, HIV infection, etc. are spreading in addition to affecting water, soil and environment at large in the country. Also the burning of plastic and untreated pharmaceutical products emits extremely toxic gases like dioxin and furans, which further add up to the environment pollution.[68]

The healthcare waste generated at scattered, small sources is equally hazardous. These sources include home-based healthcare (e.g. dialysis), and illicit drug use (usually intravenous). Many of the dangers or hazards associated with biomedical wastes are hidden. Injuries may not occur right away but might build up or lie dormant in the body system for years like hepatitis B and C and cancers. Hence, all suspected unknown substances should be considered hazardous.[66]

HAZARDS OF BIOMEDICAL/HEALTHCARE WASTE

About 75 to 90 percent of the waste produced by healthcare providers is nonhazardous "general waste" comparable to domestic waste.

Types of Hazards

The exposure to hazardous healthcare waste can result into:

1. Infection
2. Physical injuries
3. Chemical toxicity
4. Radioactivity hazards
5. Genotoxicity and cytotoxicity
6. Public sensitivity.

Infection: Portal of entry of the infectious agent into the body may be:

a. Through a puncture, abrasion, or cut in the skin
b. Through mucous membranes
c. By inhalation and ingestion.

Most Common infections, which can result from mishandling of hospital/healthcare waste, are:

1. Gastroenteric infections through feces and/or vomit (*Salmonella, Shigella spp., Vibrio cholerae*, Helminthes; Hepatitis A).
2. Respiratory infections through inhaled secretions; saliva (*Mycobacterium tuberculosis*; measles virus; *Streptococcus pneumoniae*).
3. Genital infections (*Neisseria gonorrhoeae*; herpes virus).
4. Ocular infections through eye secretions (herpes virus).
5. Skin infection through pus (Streptococcus spp.).
6. AIDS through blood and sexual secretions (HIV).
7. Meningitis through cerebrospinal fluid (*Neisseria meningitides*).
8. Septicemia and bacteremia through blood (*Staphylococcus aureus, Enterococcus, Enterobacter, Klebsiella and Streptococcus*).
9. Viral hepatitis B and C through blood and body fluids (hepatitis B and C viruses).
10. Hemorrhagic fevers through body fluids (Junin, Lassa, Ebola and Marburg viruses).

Physical injuries: Can be attributed to sharps, chemicals and explosive agents.

Chemical toxicity: Various chemicals and pharmaceutical drugs which are used in hospitals for different purposes, have potentially harmful effects. These effects may be due to the physical properties and chemical nature of these products. They may result in toxicity by both acute or chronic exposure and injuries like burns.

Radioactivity hazards: The exposure to radioactive waste may cause headache, dizziness, vomiting, tissue damage, genotoxicity, etc.

Genotoxicity and cytotoxicity: Many cytotoxic drugs are extremely irritant. Their direct contact with skin and eyes also produces harmful local effects. Many pharmaceutical drugs are carcinogenic and mutagenic; secondary neoplasia is known to be associated with chemotherapy.

Public sensitivity.[6]

Persons at Risk

Every individual who is exposed to hazardous healthcare waste is potentially at risk, including those within healthcare establishments that generate hazardous waste, and those outside these sources who either handle such waste or are exposed to it as a consequence of careless management. The main groups at risk are the following:

- Doctors, dentists, nurses, healthcare assistants and hospital maintenance personnel (Fig. 5.1)

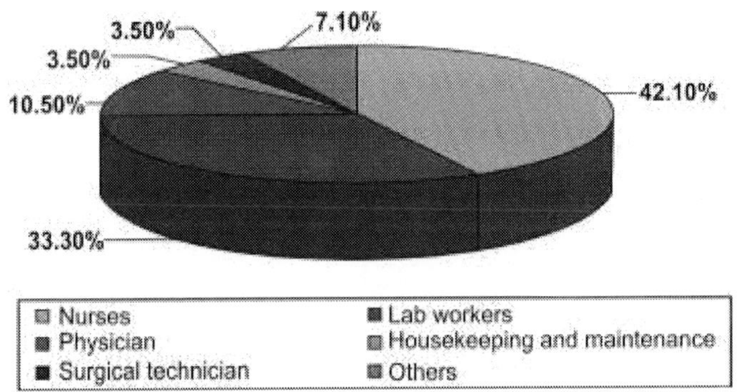

Fig. 5.1: Pie chart showing statistics about healthcare workers who acquired HIV/ AIDS at work during 1981–2002

Source: *Worker Chartbook 2004 NIOSH Publication No. 2004-146*
(For color version see Plate 1)

- Patients in healthcare establishments or receiving home care and visitors at these sites
- Workers in allied support services to healthcare establishments such as laundries, waste handling and transportation
- Workers in waste disposal facilities (such as landfills or incinerators), including scavengers.

Hazards from Infectious Waste and Sharps (Figs 5.2 and 5.3)

Transmission of Human Immunodeficiency Virus (HIV) and hepatitis viruses B and C via healthcare waste has emerged as a

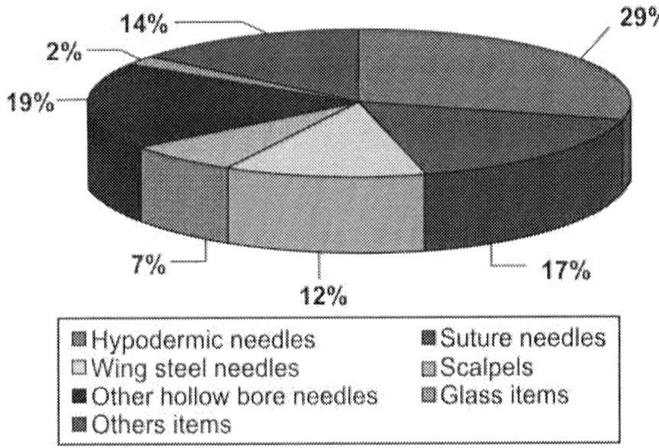

Fig. 5.2: Statistics about medical devices associated with percutaneous injuries during 1995–2000

Source: *Worker Health Chartbook 2004 NIOSH Publication No. 2004-146*
(For color version see Plate 1)

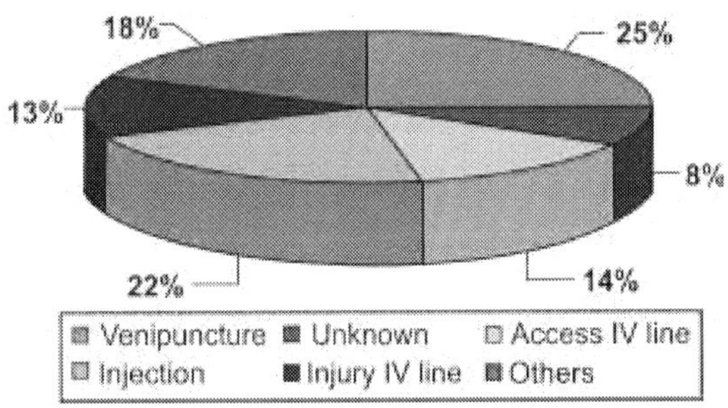

Fig. 5.3: Statistics about medical procedures involving hollow-bore needles associated with percutaneous injuries during 1995–2000

Source: *Worker Health Chartbook 2004 NIOSH Publication No. 2004-146*
(For color version see Plate 2)

serious threat to public. These viruses are generally transmitted through injuries from sharps contaminated with human blood.[66]

The practice of reusing the syringes/needles is still going on in rural India. Hence, putting an innumerable and unrecorded number of persons at risk.[100]

The evolution and spread of bacteria resistant to antibiotics and chemical disinfectants may also be related to poorly managed healthcare waste. For example, plasmids from laboratory strains contained in healthcare waste can be transferred to indigenous bacteria via the waste disposal system.

Contaminated sharps (particularly hypodermic needles) are probably the most acute potential hazards to health because:

1. Sharps, if they are contaminated with pathogens, may not only cause cuts and punctures, but also infect these wounds.
2. The infections that may be transmitted by subcutaneous introduction of the causative agent, e.g. viral blood infections, as hypodermic needles are often contaminated with patient's blood.[66]

Chances of infection to healthcare worker from an infected syringe have been estimated are as follows: hepatitis B: 30 percent; hepatitis C: 1.8 percent; HIV: 0.3 percent.[99]

Do You Know?

- Just 0.1 ml of blood is enough to cause infection in case of HIV and 0.00004 ml of blood may be enough to cause an infection in case of HBV.
- The quantity of infectious virus in plasma or serum of HIV infected individuals is estimated to be 10 to 15 infectious particles (ip)/ml with the highest levels of 10^4 ip/ml in patients with AIDS. A small amount of freely circulating virus in the blood could explain the low risk of infection following a needlestick injury compared to that of HBV, which is present in infected individuals at 10^9 ip/ml. In other body fluids like tears, saliva and ear secretions the virus titer is one tenth or one hundredth of the titer in blood.
- Also HBV is more viable than HIV.
- In March 2000, it was estimated that 0.6 to 0.8 million needle stick injuries and other percutaneous injuries occur annually among healthcare workers.

- Occupational Safety and Heath Administration (OSHA), USA, estimated that 8 million workers in the healthcare industry and related occupations worldwide are at risk of occupational exposure to blood-borne pathogens[81]
- According to WHO (2000) injections with contaminated syringes caused 21 million hepatitis B virus infections (32% of all new infections); 2 million hepatitis C virus infections (40% of all new infections) and 2,60,000 HIV infections (5% of all new infections)[99]
- In India, 16 billion injections are given per year that makes the count to 45 million per day.[30]

Impacts of Infectious Waste and Sharps

Apart from spreading serious infections like HIV/AIDS, HBV and HCV to healthcare workers (especially nurses), contaminated sharps (particularly hypodermic needles) can put at risk other hospital workers, waste management operators outside hospitals, and scavengers on waste disposal sites.

Certain infections may spread through other media or caused by more resistance strains/agents. Such infections may pose a significant risk to hospital's patients and to the general public. So another impact is spread of epidemics due to uncontrolled discharge of sewage from hospital down the drains to municipal sanitary sewer.

Hazards from Chemical and Pharmaceutical Waste

Most of the chemicals and pharmaceuticals used in healthcare establishments are hazardous (e.g. toxic, genotoxic, corrosive, flammable, reactive, explosive, shock-sensitive). Their intoxication can occur either by acute or by chronic exposure. The intoxication and injuries (including burns) are potential hazards. Intoxication can result from:

- Inhalation
- Ingestion
- Absorption of a chemical or pharmaceutical through the skin or the mucous membranes.

Contact with flammable, corrosive, or reactive chemicals, (e.g. formaldehyde and other volatile substances) can cause injuries to the skin, the eyes, or the mucous membranes of the airways, the most common injuries being the chemical burns. These substances are commonly present in small quantities in health-care waste; larger quantities may be found when unwanted or outdated chemicals and pharmaceuticals are disposed off.

Disinfectants are used in large quantities and are often corrosive. When their chemical residues are discharged into the sewage system, they may affect the operation of biological sewage treatment plants adversely and have toxic effects on the natural ecosystems of receiving waters. Pharmaceutical residues, including antibiotics and other drugs, heavy metals such as mercury, phenols and its derivatives, disinfectants and antiseptics may pose similar challenges.

Impacts of Chemical and Pharmaceutical Waste

Although chemical or pharmaceutical waste from hospitals has not been related to widespread illness among the general public, extensive intoxication caused by industrial chemical waste is a well known fact.[66] Fish in Sutlej river in Punjab die in masses due to discharge of untreated industrial waste into the river which has raised many eyebrows.[4]

Hazards From Genotoxic Waste

The severity of the hazards of genotoxic waste is governed by a combination of two factors:

1. Substance toxicity itself.
2. The extent and duration of exposure.

Exposure to genotoxic substances in healthcare occurs during:

a. The preparation of particular drug/chemicals
b. Treatment with particular drugs or chemicals.
c. Handling and disposal.

The main pathways of exposure are:

A. Inhalation: Inhalation of dust or aerosols.
B. Ingestion:
- Ingestion of food accidentally contaminated with cytotoxic drugs, chemicals, or waste
- Ingestion as a result of bad practice, such as mouth pipetting.

C. Contact:

- Absorption through the skin.
- Contact with the body fluids and secretions of patients undergoing chemotherapy.

The cytotoxic effect of many antineoplastic drugs is cell cycle-specific, targeting specific intracellular processes such as DNA synthesis and mitosis. However, other antineoplastic drugs, e.g. alkylating agents are not phase specific. They exert their cytotoxic effect at any point in the cell cycle. Many cytotoxic drugs (Table 5.1) are extremely irritant. Their direct contact with skin and eyes also produces harmful local and systemic effects such as dermatitis, nausea, headache, dizziness, etc.

Impacts of Genotoxic Waste

An increased risk of abortion and increased urinary levels of mutagenic compounds were noted in workers who handled these antineoplastc drugs. The exposure of personnel cleaning hospital urinals is found to be more than that of nurses and pharmacists because these individuals were less aware of the danger and took fewer precautions.

Hazards from Radioactive Waste

The type and extent of exposure determines the type of disease caused by radioactive waste. It can range from minor symptoms

Table 5.1: Cytotoxic drugs hazardous to eyes and skin

Alkylating agents	
Vesicant drugs:	Aclarubicin, chlormethine, cisplatin, mitomycin
Irritant drugs:	Carmustine, cyclophosphamide, dacarbazine, ifosfamide, melphalan, streptozocin, thiotepa
Intercalating agents	
Vesicant drugs:	Amsacrine, dactinomycin, daunorubicin, doxorubicin, epirubicin, pirarubicin, zorubicin
Irritant drugs:	Mitoxantrone
Vinca alkaloids and derivatives	
Vesicant drugs:	Vinblastine, vincristine, vindesine, vinorelbine
Epipodophyllotoxins	
Irritant drugs:	Teniposide

Source: *Pruss A, Giroult E, Rushbrook, Safe Management of Waste from Healthcare activities (WHO).*

like headache, dizziness, and vomit to more serious problems. Because radioactive waste is genotoxic, it may affect genetic material. Handling of highly active sources may cause more severe injuries such as destruction of tissue, necessitating amputation of body parts, e.g. certain sealed sources from diagnostic instruments. So these should be handled with the utmost care.

The exposure to low-activity waste may arise from contamination of external surfaces of containers or improper mode or duration of waste storage. Healthcare workers or waste-handling or cleaning personnel exposed to this radioactivity are at potential risk.

Impacts of Radioactive Waste

Improper disposal of nuclear therapeutic materials have lead to several accidents in history. A large number of persons are presently suffering from the results of exposure while many of them go unreported. The other sources of accidental exposure to ionizing radiations in healthcare settings have resulted from unsafe operation of X-ray apparatus, improper handling of radiotherapy solutions, or inadequate control of radiotherapy.[66] Indiscriminate disposal of radioactive waste in general waste stream may create some serious and life-threatening situation. One such accidental exposure to high activity radioactive waste in New Delhi in April 2010 left five persons critically ill.[88]

Public Sensitivity

Quite apart from fear of health hazards, the general public is very sensitive about the visual impact of *anatomical waste*, which is recognizable human body parts, including fetuses. It is unacceptable to dispose of this anatomical waste inappropriately, such as on a landfill where it is visible to public or approachable to stray animals. In some cultures, especially in Asia, it is a religious belief that human body parts be returned to a patient's family, in tiny "coffins," to be buried in cemeteries.[66] The Muslim culture, too, generally requires that body parts are buried in cemeteries while Hindus burn them.

Need for Disposal of Biomedical Waste

It is rightly said that 'Cleanliness is next to Godliness'. Proper biomedical waste management is the mainstay of hospital cleanliness, hospital hygiene and maintenance activities.[20] Healthcare waste poses a threat to health and lives of patients, staff and community through direct contact or through environment pollution[39] (Fig. 6.1).

Effective and efficient methods of biomedical waste disposal should be employed to prevent such harms. This requires a huge investment in terms of money, material, manpower and machinery. Then question arises as to what is the need or rationale for such expenditure? The rationale is health, ethical and environmental.

HEALTH REASONS

- Injuries may lead to infections to healthcare workers and waste handlers
- Hospital acquired infection can spread due to poor practices of infection control and waste management

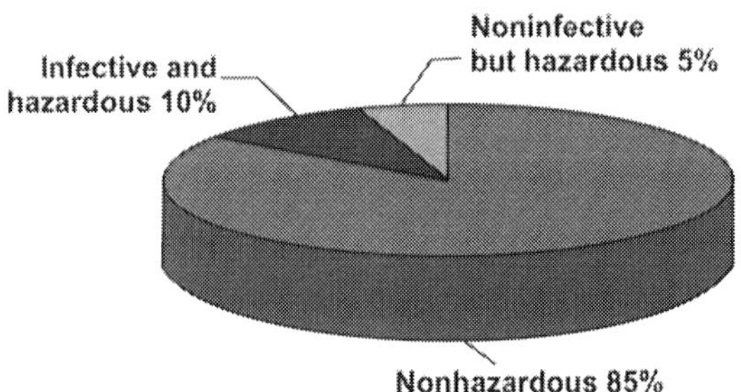

Fig. 6.1: Pie chart showing different categories of hospital waste[70]

- Risk of infection for waste handlers, scavengers and general public in the vicinity of hospitals
- Risk due to drugs and hazardous chemicals to persons handling wastes at each level
- "Disposable" items being repacked and marketed by unscrupulous elements without any disinfection
- Repacking and resale of discarded drugs
- Risk of air, water and soil pollution due to waste itself or its defective disposal, e.g. incineration generates emission of gases like furan, dioxin, hydrochloric acid (HCl) and fly ash[20]
- Tubercle bacilli spores remain suspended in the air and can spread tuberculosis
- Soil may be polluted by tetanus spores
- Pollution of water and food by biological agents results in alimentary infections like typhoid, cholera, infective hepatitis, polio, dysentery, ascariasis and hookworm diseases, etc.
- Various vectors of disease transmission such as worms and pests breed on the wastes, e.g. mosquitoes transmit malaria and filaria
- Hospital acquired infections like AIDS, hepatitis B and C, etc.[101]

ETHICAL ASPECTS

It is the moral duty of healthcare workers to prevent hospitals from becoming centers of disease rather than center of cure. The rationale of biomedical waste management includes:

- Raising awareness on public health and environment hazards associated with inappropriate segregation, collection, storage, transport, handling, treatment and disposal of healthcare waste
- Providing information on hazards and sound management practices of healthcare waste for the policy making, development and improvement of legislation and technical guidelines
- Identifying safe, efficient, sustainable, economic and culturally acceptable waste management practices and technologies and enabling the participants to identify the systems according to their particular needs

- Enabling managers of healthcare establishments to develop their waste management plans
- Enabling course participants to develop training programs.[67]

ENVIRONMENTAL REASONS

As mentioned before, biomedical waste can cause air, water and soil pollution.

Although pollution cannot be eliminated completely, efforts can be done to minimize it.

Air pollution: It is of three types:
1. Biological
2. Chemical
3. Radioactive.

Biological

i. Air pollution inside the premises

Pathogens or their spores can enter and remain suspended in the air inside the building of the healthcare establishment for a prolonged period. This can result in nosocomial infections or occupational health hazards. This puts healthcare workers, patients as well as their attendants at risk of contracting airborne infections.

Indoor air pollution can be attributed to:
- **Poor ventilation:** Improper planning and faulty air conditioning results in poor circulation of air within the rooms. So design of the building has an important role to play in maintaining proper ventilation.
- **Use of chemicals:** Disinfectants, fumigants, etc. release acidic or hazardous gases or vapors into the air.

ii. Outdoor air pollution

When untreated waste is transported outside the healthcare establishment, or dumped openly, pathogens in the waste can contaminate drinking water, foodstuff, soil, etc. These may also remain in the ambient air and cause airborne diseases in animals and human beings.

Chemical Pollutants

Chemical pollutants of air come from two major sources—open burning and incinerators. Open burning of biomedical waste is the most harmful practice. The plastics and hazardous materials present in the waste generate oxides of sulfur and nitrogen, carbon dioxide, dioxin, furans, suspended particulate matter, etc. When inhaled, these harmful chemicals can cause respiratory diseases. Out of these, dioxins and furans are carcinogenic.

Radioactive Emissions

Small quantities of radioactive gas are generated during research and radioimmunoassay activities. The clinical application of Kr^{85} and Xe^{133} are the principal sources of gaseous radioactive waste.

Water Pollution

Improper disposal of biomedical waste, for example, dumping in low-lying areas, or into lakes and water bodies, can lead to severe water pollution. Water can be polluted by biologicals, chemicals or radioactive substances. The pathogens and harmful chemicals (heavy metals) present in the waste can leach out and contaminate the ground water or surface water.

Eutrophication: Algal brooms over surface of water bodies. This occurs mainly because of excess nutrient leachates, e.g. nitrates and phosphates from landfills. Water pollution can alter parameters such as pH, Biological Oxygen Demand (BOD). Dioxins have been reported from water bodies near incinerator plants where they enter the water body from the air. Radioactive effluents also pollute water.

Land Pollution

As all types of biomedical waste is finally disposed off on the land, land pollution is inevitable. Even liquid effluent after treatment is spread on land. However, if treated in a proper way, pollution can be minimized to a large extent. The main sources of soil pollution from biomedical waste are infectious waste, discarded medicines, chemicals waste ash and other waste generated during treatment processes. Heavy metals present in the waste such as cadmium, lead, mercury, etc. will get absorbed by plants and can then enter the food chain. Excessive amounts of trace nutrient elements and heavy metals in soil are harmful to crops, animals and human beings. Open dumping of biomedical waste is the greatest cause for land pollution and landfilling is also not a totally safe method.[5]

CHAPTER 7

Waste Minimization

DEFINITION

Waste minimization is the process and policy of reducing the amount of waste produced by a person or a society.[33]

NEED FOR WASTE MINIMIZATION

Only 15 percent of the hospital generated waste is hazardous, and rest of 85 percent is nonhazardous as per World Health Organization (WHO) but when these are mixed, a huge stock of waste is generated which needs disposal. This carries a lot many disadvantages such as increased risk to the personal in direct indirect contact with waste, increased environmental hazards, increased cost of handling and disposal. To overcome such challenges, it is advised to minimize the waste as much as possible.[66]

It is the duty of the hospital authorities to identify and quantify the waste generated. Effective measures should be taken to reduce the amount of waste by controlling the demand/inventory, wastage of consumable items and breakages, etc. Another option is recycling of certain wastes such as paper, glassware, plastic material, etc. however after proper cleaning and disinfection.[84]

As far as possible, healthcare establishments should encourage purchase of reusable items made of glass and metal. Substitute PVC (Polyvinyl Chloride) plastic items with non PVC items. Procedures and policies for proper management of waste generated should be adopted. Meticulous segregation is the key to minimize the quantity of waste to be treated. Effective and sound recycling policy for plastic recycling should be made and implemented, and authorized manufactures should be consulted wherever need be.[20]

ADVANTAGES OF WASTE MINIMIZATION

- Reduced potential for exposures of employees, patients, visitors and waste management personnel to hazards associated with wastes in terms of health and safety
- Reduced volume and toxicity of unavoidable waste
- Improved transportation, storage, treatment and disposal of waste
- Proper containment of hazardous materials
- Prompt removal of hazardous materials from the workplace.
- Long-term economic benefit.[72]

How to do Waste Minimization?

Apart from protecting people and the environment, waste minimization can save hospitals a great deal of money in the long run. Waste can be minimized by various methods:

1. **Source reduction:** The amount of waste generated at the source itself can be minimized through product substitution, technology change and good operating practices. By changing the purchasing policies and product substitution, toxicity of the waste generated can also be reduced.[82] The methods that can be adopted are:
   - Prevent wastage of products in nursing and cleaning activities, etc.
   - Prefer physical cleaning methods over chemical ones (e.g. autoclaving instead of chemical disinfection)
   - Select supplies that are less wasteful or less hazardous
   - Centralize the purchasing of hazardous chemicals at hospital level.[67]
2. **Resource recovery and recycling:** The majority of waste from healthcare facilities is same as that of an office, e.g. paper, cardboard and food wastes. Healthcare establishment can implement very simple programs that divert these materials from the solid waste stream, lowering disposal costs.[81] Wherever applicable, recycling should be adopted as a method of disposal and recycled material should be bought and used.[67]

However, recycling is usually not practiced by healthcare facilities, except for the recovery of silver from fixing-baths used in processing of X-ray films. Recycling of materials such as metals, paper, glass, and plastics can generate revenues for the healthcare facility–either through reduced disposal costs or through payments made by the recycling company.[66]

Packaging materials that can be recycled include:

- Paper and cardboard
- Plastic wrappings
- Metal containers
- Glass.

Consideration should be given to segregation of materials that could be recycled, considering the market opportunities.[67]

3. **Educating the staff:** It is mandatory to train the nursing and housekeeping staff in the methods of proper segregation of waste. They must be educated about the different categories of waste so that they may be able to distinguish between infectious and noninfectious waste. This has been discussed in detail in chapter on **'Training of Healthcare Workers.'**
4. **Composting organic waste:** Composting is a type of recycling. Organic waste, e.g. vegetable food scraps, is mixed with a nitrogen source and provided with air and water. After some time, the waste changes into compost, that is used in lawns, gardens or farms to add nutrients and texture to the soil.[82]

A FEW EXAMPLES OF WASTE MINIMIZATION PROCEDURES

Minimizing Chemical Waste

Chemotherapy and Antineoplastic Chemicals

- Centralize chemotherapy compounding location
- Optimize the size of the drug container while purchasing
- Reduce the volume to be used
- Employ effective spill clean up procedure
- Segregate the wastes from other wastes
- Return the outdated drugs to the manufacturer.

Formaldehyde

- Minimize the concentration/strength of formaldehyde solutions
- Minimize the waste from cleaning of dialysis machines and reverse osmosis units
- Capture the waste formaldehyde
- Reuse in pathology, autopsy labs, etc.

Solvents

- Minimize the volume requirement
- For tests involving solvent fixation, use premixed kits
- Recover used solvents through distillation
- For routine tests, always use calibrated solvent dispensers.

Photographic Chemicals

- Return spare developer to the manufacturer
- Keep developer and fixer cans covered to prevent evaporation.

Waste Anesthetic Gases

- Minimize the wastage through leakage by employing proper maintenance.

Toxic Corrosives and Miscellaneous Chemicals

- Avoid spills
- Neutralize the acidic wastes by mixing with basic wastes
- Use compounds, cleaning agents, etc. with lesser toxicity
- Inspect and properly maintain ethylene oxide sterilizers
- Reuse, return and recycle containers
- For laundry equipments, use automated system
- Use physical cleaning methods instead of chemical ones.[44]

Reuse

Various equipments used for diagnosis, treatment and other activities in healthcare establishments can be reused, if they are designed for this purpose and if they can withstand the process of sterilization. Items that may be reused include metallic and glassware such as certain sharps, i.e. scalpels, hypodermic needles and syringes, containers, glass bottles, etc. After use, collect these separately from disposable items, wash (hypodermic needles especially), and sterilize by one of the following processes.

Thermal Sterilization

- *Dry heat sterilization*: Exposure to 160°C for 120 minutes or 170°C for 60 minutes in a "Hot air oven".
- *Steam sterilization*: Exposure to saturated steam at 121°C for 30 minutes in an autoclave.

Cold Sterilization/Chemical Sterilization

- **Ethylene oxide:** Ethylene oxide is a very hazardous chemical. So sterilization in a 'gas-sterilizer' should be carried out only by highly trained and adequately protected technical personnel.

The procedure involves exposure of the infected matter to ethylene oxide for 3 to 8 hours, at 50 to 60°C, in a reactor tank. (The so-called "gas-sterilizer" tank should be dry before injection of the ethylene oxide).

- **Glutaraldehyde:** This process is safer for the operators than ethylene oxide, but is less efficient microbiologically. Exposure to a glutaraldehyde solution for 30 minutes is recommended.

Plastic syringes and catheters should be discarded and not to be reused. Pins, needles or seeds of long-half life radionuclides used for radiotherapy may be reused after sterilization.[66]

Waste Segregation and Labeling

WASTE SEGREGATION

Segregation is defined as "separation of different types of wastes by sorting or the systematic separation of biomedical waste into designated categories."[101]

The concepts of waste minimization and green purchasing (i.e. environment friendly purchasing) must be considered before charting out waste segregation plan. The waste that cannot be minimized should be segregated at the source into the relevant categories for disposal. Color-coded of waste segregation renders protection to workers, minimizes harm to and the environment as well as reduces the cost of disposal.[37]

Need for Segregation of BMW at Source

- If proper segregation of the waste is not done at source, the biomedical waste and the municipal waste of the hospital might get mixed up
- Waste segregation is the backbone of waste minimization and efficient and meticulous waste collection, transportation, treatment and disposal
- The unsegregated BMW may put human and the animal lives in danger
- The unsegregated BMW may hamper the entire process of the BMW treatment.[95]

How Does Segregation Help?

- It prevents illegal reuse of certain components of healthcare waste like used syringes, needles and other plastics
- It provides an opportunity for recycling certain components of healthcare waste like plastics after proper and thorough

disinfection. This recycled plastic material can be used for non-foodgrade applications. Recycling can also generate revenues

- The biodegradable general waste can be composted within the hospital premises and can be used for gardening purposes
- Segregation reduces the cost of treatment and disposal.[9]

Segregation is the most vital step in effective healthcare waste management. It ensures correct routes for disposal, personnel safety and minimal environmental harm. Segregation of health-care waste should be based on the final treatment/disposal requirements.

Segregation should be done under the supervision of the waste producer close to the point of generation, that is, at the bedside, in the ward, in the theater, in the delivery room, in the laboratory, etc. It must be carried out by the person who generates the waste, e.g. the doctor or the specialist, the nurse. This activity secures the waste immediately and avoids dangerous secondary sorting. Correct and efficient segregation requires a dedicated rigorous training and education of employees, supervisors and managers, and policies drafted after considering these points.

The same segregation system should be uniformly practiced throughout the whole country. The segregation must be practiced from the point of generation to the point of final disposal including all storage and transportation methods.

Segregated wastes of different categories should be collected in identifiable containers. To ensure proper procedure, instructions for waste segregation and identification should be placed at each waste collection point.

A preferred system of labeling and coding of packaging for identifying biomedical and healthcare waste categories is by sorting the waste into color-coded bags or containers (Fig. 8.1). Internationally recognized symbols and signs are essential for the safe handling and disposal of waste. The color coding, the symbols and signs should be included in the waste management instructions and should be displayed appropriately, e.g. a poster on the wall at the waste collection points.

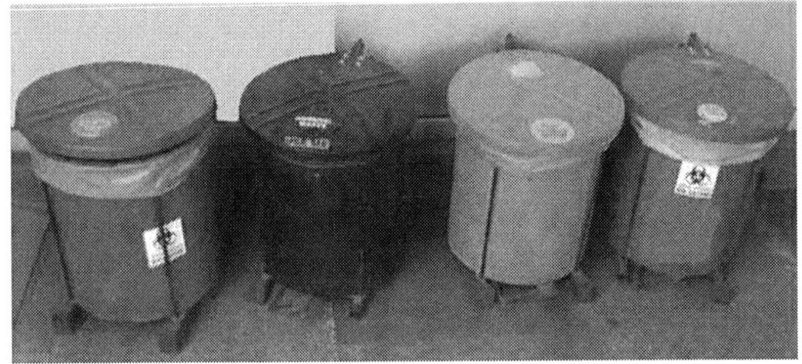

Fig. 8.1: Color-coded containers
(For color version see Plate 2)

Clinical and sanitary personnel must ensure that the waste bags are sealed and removed when they are less than three-quarters full.[78]

The segregation of biomedical waste should be carefully examined because facility standard operating procedures for segregation of BMW directly influence the type and cost of BMW treatment. The waste has to be kept segregated in an appropriate container or bag as per its category. A few essential properties of such containers or bags are as follows:

- It should not leak
- The container should have a cover (preferably foot controlled)
- It must have the capacity to contain the designed volume and bear the weight of the waste without any damage
- When a bag or container is 3/4th full, it must be securely sealed and an appropriate label has to be attached.

An adequate symbol must be displayed for each type of BMW, according to their code:

1. Pathological waste
2. Infectious waste
3. Sharps
4. Chemical waste
5. Pharmaceutical waste
6. Genotoxic waste
7. Radioactive waste
8. Waste with high content of heavy metals.[8]

Cautions

- Never compact biomedical waste at the point of origin
- Biomedical waste should be removed from its container or point of origin only by a licensed biomedical waste disposal firm
- Never mix biomedical waste with radioactive or hazardous chemical waste.[29]

Role of Waste Segregation

- It is the mainstay of waste minimization
- It is must for effective waste management
- It improves protection of public health.

REQUIREMENTS FOR WASTE SEGREGATION

- It should be undertaken on the basis of the types of waste listed in the definition for biomedical and healthcare waste
- Each healthcare institution should prepare and follow a waste plan
- It should be based on specific ultimate/final treatment and disposal requirements
- It should be carried out under the supervision of or by the waste producer himself at source
- It should be applied uniformly all over the country
- It should be started from production site and maintained till disposal
- It should be initiated at the source only, i.e. in the ward at the patient's bedside, in the operation theater, in the laboratory or other areas in the hospital where the waste is generated
- It should be easy for the medical and auxiliary staff to implement
- It should be safe to practice
- It should ensure that infectious healthcare waste does not mingle with the domestic waste flow
- The medical and auxiliary staff should be thorough with the waste segregation measures
- It should be regularly monitored to ensure that the procedures are being practiced accurately
- It should ensure that correct disposal routes are being taken and personnel safety is maintained.[78]

SIGNIFICANCE

Only a small proportion of the wastes generated at a healthcare or similar facility are actually biomedical wastes. Segregation minimizes the amount of waste requiring special handling and disposal procedures and reduces the overall costs of waste disposal as the entire waste stream does not have to be treated as biomedical waste. Waste segregation separates infectious and hazardous waste from general waste, thereby reducing not only the risks, but also the cost of handling, treatment and disposal.

PERSONS RESPONSIBLE FOR SEGREGATION

Segregation of wastes takes very little extra time and is not costly. That is the reason why waste segregation must be done at the point of its generation, i.e. the source. According to Disposal of Biomedical Waste (Handling and Management) Rules, 1998, segregation of biomedical waste is the responsibility of the generator of the waste, i.e. the persons in any healthcare establishment who generate or produce wastes (doctors, nurses, paramedical staff, patients and their caretakers).[101] The reason behind this principle is that healthcare workers are:

- Well aware about materials used and their purpose.
- Know the items, materials used on infectious patients, laboratory experiments, etc.
- Know which chemicals, pharmaceuticals or cytotoxics were used.
- Wear the proper Personal Protective Equipments (PPEs).
- Trained and have expertise for waste disposal.

PROCEDURE FOR SEGREGATION

A. Segregation of biomedical waste should be done in accordance with schedule II of BMW Rules, 1998 (see page 21).
B. The radioactive waste produced within hospitals are generally segregated as follows (Table 8.1).

Table 8.1: Categories of packages for radioactive waste

Conditions		
Maximum radiation level at a distance of 1 m from the external surface of the package	*Maximum radiation level at any point on the external surface*	*Category*
Not more than 0.0005 mSv/h	Not more than 0.005 mSv/h	I-White
More than 0.0005 mSv/h but Not more than 0.01 mSv/h	More than 0.005 mSv/h but not more than 0.5 mSv/h	II-Yellow
More than 0.01 mSv/h but Not more than 0.1 mSv/h	More than 0.5 mSv/h but not more than 2 mSv/h	III-Yellow

Source: *Pruss A, Giroult E, Rushbrook, Safe Management of Waste from Healthcare activities (WHO).*

C. General waste should be categorized as follows:

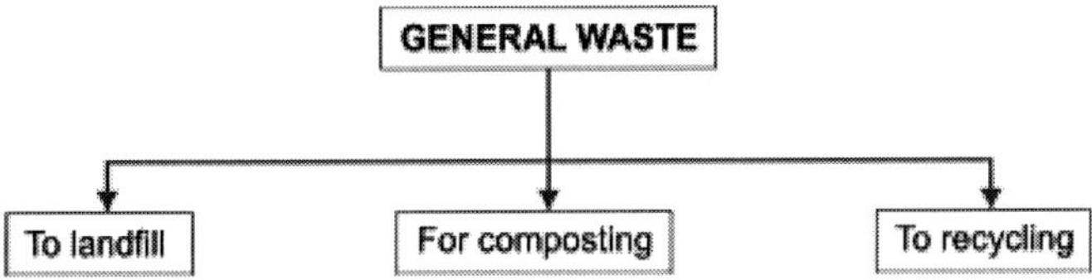

1. Waste that will go to landfill
2. Waste that can be sent for compost, e.g. flowers and vegetables scraps
3. Waste that can be recycled for, e.g. paper, cardboard, aluminum cans, plastics.[46]

RULES FOR SEGREGATION

1. Segregation and labeling of wastes should be carried out at source. The biohazard symbol must be clearly visible on the bins used for collection of biomedical waste.
2. Color coding for containers and various types of waste is must for meticulous segregation. Locations for containers or bag holders should be determined on the basis of particular

categories of waste generated. Pamphlets/charts of instructions for waste segregation and identification should be pasted at each waste collection point as a reminder for the staff. When the containers three-quarters full, they should be removed.
3. If nonhazardous and hazardous wastes are accidentally mixed, the entire mixture should be treated as hazardous waste.
4. Staff should never attempt correction of errors of segregation, e.g. removing items from a bag/container after disposal, or putting one bag inside another bag of a different color.[39]

Advantages of Color-coded Waste Containers

A. It makes it easy for the staff to properly segregate wastes.
B. It renders the various types of wastes/contents of the bin easily identifiable.
C. The potential hazards of these wastes can be easily identified.
D. Various treatment and disposal requirements for these wastes can be readily selected.[46]

Note

- Whenever possible, highly infectious waste should be immediately sterilized by autoclaving. It is recommended that these wastes should be packaged in bags compatible with the autoclave, i.e. red bags
- Low-level radioactive infectious waste, (e.g. swabs, syringes used for diagnostic or therapeutic purposes) may be collected in same yellow bags or containers for infectious waste, if these are to be incinerated.[66]

ADVANTAGES OF SEGREGATION

Following are the advantages of proper segregation of wastes:
1. It minimizes the amount of hazardous waste
2. It saves costs for healthcare establishments
3. It reduces occupational health hazards to healthcare workers
4. It prevents cross-contamination of various wastes, thus improves infection control.[46]

CONTAINERS FOR WASTE COLLECTION

Good quality plastics or other strong material such as metals should be used for fabrication of all types of waste containers. The inner and outer surfaces of these containers should be smooth to prevent dirt/dust sticking in indentations. They may or may not be lined with nonchlorinated plastic liners. They should always be kept closed. For potentially infected wastes, 2 percent bleach solution (freshly prepared twice daily) should be put in the waste container and the waste should be put in the container having this solution. The quantity of waste in each of the waste containers should be weighed prior to evacuating the container into the final onsite disposal, and a log should be maintained.[53]

The containers should be labeled in such a way that they are easily identifiable and recognizable to all staff. They should be color-coded and clearly marked according to the Biomedical Waste (Management and Handling) Rules, 1998.

Incinerable healthcare wastes should be disposed in 'non-polyvinyl chloride' plastic bags. For biomedical waste storage, mobile garbage bins with capacity of 50, 60, 120, 240 or 660 liters are ideal. The containers used should be nonreactive with any of the wastes.[46]

Types of Containers

Reusable Containers (Fig. 8.2)

These containers (e.g. plastic bins) must be made of rigid plastic and able to withstand repeated exposure to the common cleaning agents. They should be color-coded according to the type of waste for which they are intended, and must be labeled with the biohazard symbol.

Reusable waste containers should be carefully inspected for holes or leaks each time they are emptied and their color-coding and labeling renewed, whenever necessary. If holes or leaks are found, these must be repaired or the waste container replaced. If waste materials leak or spill within the containers, reusable waste containers must be disinfected regularly to prevent odors and contamination as soon as possible.

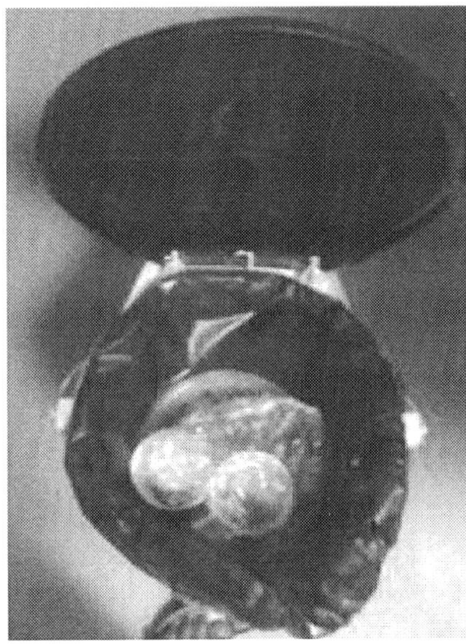

Fig. 8.2: Reusable container

Note: Containers designated for single use should never be reused.

Sharps Containers (Fig. 8.3)

Sharps containers should be made up of metal or high density plastic which makes them puncture proof and impermeable under normal conditions of use and handling, so that they safely retain not only the sharps, but also any residual liquids from syringes. The containers may be color-coded but must be labeled with the biohazard symbol and have tightly secured lids. If the proposed treatment process for sharps containers is autoclaving, they must remain functionally intact at high autoclaving temperatures.[54] Where plastic or metal containers are unavailable or too costly, containers made of dense cardboard are recommended.[66]

Other useful features for sharps container include:

- A fill line up to 3/4th of its capacity
- Should be tamper proof, (i.e. difficult to open/break) to prevent unauthorized persons from removing items from the container or from removing the container itself

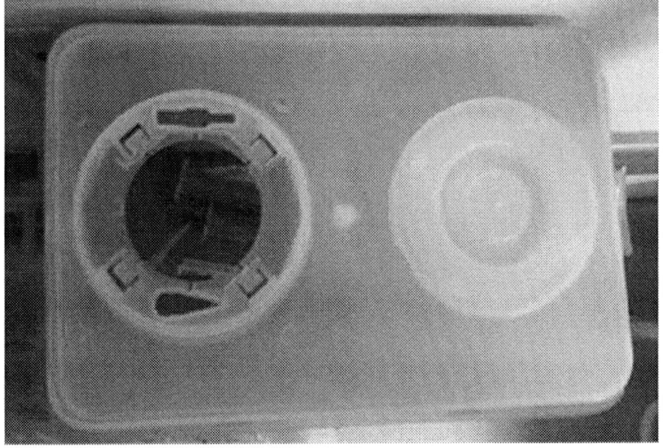

Fig. 8.3: Sharps container

- Handles that permit their safe movement before disposal
- A design that allows stacking
- A means that allows the container to be attached to mobile applications such as medication carts, treatment carts or in ambulance.

Important Points

- To minimize the chances of injury, sharps containers should be conveniently located close to the point of generation
- To prevent injuries due to overfilling, they should not be filled to more than three-quarters of their useable capacity
- Sharps should never be forced into the container.

Plastic Waste Holding Bags (Fig. 8.4)

These bags should be sturdy enough to resist puncture under conditions of use and should remain intact to the point of disposal. Each facility should thorougly test and evaluate these bags under actual conditions of use. Plastic waste-holding bags must be color-coded and labeled.

Note: For the purposes of collection and movement of waste inside the premises of healthcare establishment, appropriate thickness of plastic bags or plastic sharps wastes containers cannot be specified because physical and mechanical properties of plastic

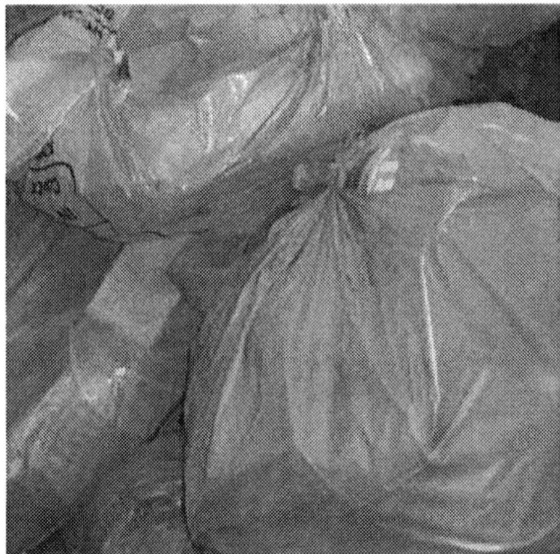

Fig. 8.4: Plastic waste holding bags

materials vary extensively. A plastic material of 25.4 micrometer thickness may be more resistant to puncture, impact and abrasion than a different plastic material of 50.8 micrometer thick film. The properties can also be affected by the manufacturing process, (i.e. extrusion or injection moulding). The, recommended thickness should be a minimum gauge of 55 micron (for low density) or 25 micron (for high density). The inner polythene bag should fit into the container with one-fourth of the polythene bag turned over the rim. The plastic bags should be made of nonhalogenated plastics, combustible, if they are destined for incineration.

Cardboard Containers

Cardboard containers should be:

- Color-coded and must be labeled with the biohazard symbol
- Rigid
- Leak-resistant
- Capable of being sealed
- Closeable.

Note: If cardboard containers are to be shipped offsite, they should be supplemented with an additional outer packaging meeting the requirements of 'transportation of dangerous goods regulations'. Alternatively, the cardboard container itself must meet the requirements of the regulations.[54]

LABELING

A tag or adhesive label should be attached to the bag/container for easy identification.[46]

Items placed in the biomedical waste bag or sharps containers are exempted from labeling when the waste bag itself is labeled.

Indelible ink shall be used to print the label and the label shall be at least three inches by five inches in size. The label shall contain the following:

- Office name
- Address
- Date when the waste was generated or packaged
- The biomedical waste symbol.

If a biohazard bag or sharps container is placed into a larger box or container, prior label for the exterior container must comply with the above information. Inner bags/containers are exempt from the labeling requirements above-mentioned.

Outer containers must be labeled with the transporter's name, address, registration number, telephone number prior to transport. The name, address, business telephone number, and registration number of the generator; "Refrigeration Required", in large print if pathological waste, cultures, or animal carcasses or body parts are included in the contents.

All packages containing biomedical waste must be visibly identifiable with biological hazard symbol and one of the following phrases: "BIOMEDICAL", "BIOHAZARDOUS WASTE," "BIOHAZARD," OR "INFECTIOUS WASTE".[25]

Labeling is must for the correct identification and hence appropriate and safe management of biomedical wastes. It acts as a warning sign to all workers, patients and the public about the existence of the waste.

All labeling and signposting should be done according to international symbols and color-coding. Also, unified system for standards or codes for hazardous wastes should be followed across the nation. Hence, adoption of correct labeling practices by both healthcare establishments and waste collection/disposal companies is essential.[46]

The following types of labeling are recommended:

- **Pathological/contaminated/infectious waste:** These wastes are disposed off in yellow plastic bags and containers. These bags/containers should be marked with the international biohazard symbol in black. The wording should comply with local regulations, e.g. "BIOHAZARD" in India.
- **Cytotoxic waste:** All containers and bags should be of yellow color that indicates wastes for destruction by incineration. They should be marked with the "C", i.e. cytotoxic hazard symbol. In addition, the words "CYTOTOXIC HAZARD" may also be used.

SCHEDULE III (SEE RULE 6)

LABEL FOR BIOMEDICAL WASTE CONTAINERS/BAGS[47]

BIOHAZARD SYMBOL जैविक परिसंकट चिन्ह	CYTOTOXIC HAZARD SYMBOL कोषिकाविष परिसंकट चिन्ह
BIOHAZARD जैविक परिसंकट	CYTOTOXIC कोषिकाविष

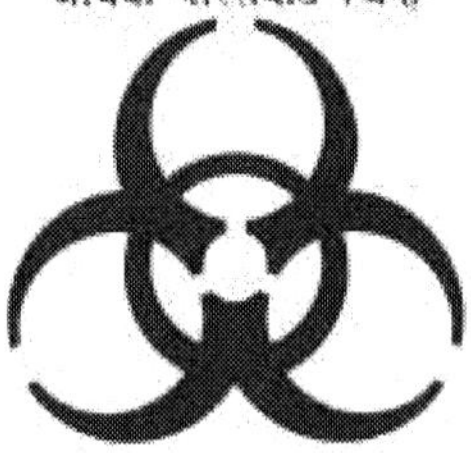

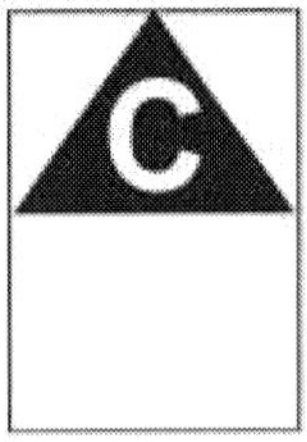

Recyclable Waste (Fig. 8.5)

1. All symbols and words must be easily identifiable and visible. The recommended size of symbol and letters is 80 mm.
2. The label must also provide the required information as mentioned in Schedule IV of BMW rules.[66]

The label should also include the following:

a. Do not overfill.
b. A fill line.
c. Words or a symbol that warns against putting hands in the container or touching waste.
d. Words that indicate that 'once a container is 3/4th full, it should be sealed securely.

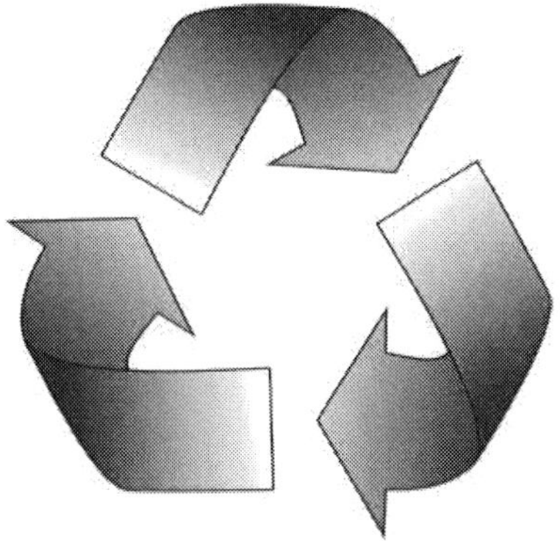

Fig. 8.5: Recyclable waste
(For color version see Plate 2)

SCHEDULE IV (SEE RULE 6)

LABEL FOR TRANSPORT OF BIOMEDICAL WASTE[52] CONTAINERS/BAGS

	Day....................Month.............
	Year..............
	Date of generation ....
Waste category no...........	
Waste class	
Waste description	
Sender's name and address	Receiver's name and address
Phone no.	Phone no. ....
Telex no.	Telex no. ....
Fax no.	Fax no. ....
Contact person	Contact person ....
In case of emergency please contact	
Name and address :	
Phone no. :	
Note :	
Label shall be nonwashable and prominently visible.	

Tagging System of Waste

The tags on the bags/bins should indicate the source of generation of waste. Apart from telling the source, tags can also act as guide to trace the areas/wards showing noncompliance to the BMW rules.[46]

CHAPTER

9 Waste Handling, Collection, Storage and Transportation

WASTE HANDLING

Waste handlers should be extra careful while handling healthcare waste. It is the most risky job to handle sharps, as sharps can cause injuries as well as infections. Untreated waste should be handled as little as possible. Sanitary staff and cleaners should always wear protective clothing including overalls or industrial aprons, heavy duty gloves and boots.[91]

Gloves

Waste handlers should use heavy duty, bright-colored rubber gloves for healthcare waste handling (Fig. 9.1). The gloves should be washed twice after handling the waste, and should be washed after every use with carbolic soap and a disinfectant. The size should fit the operator's hands.

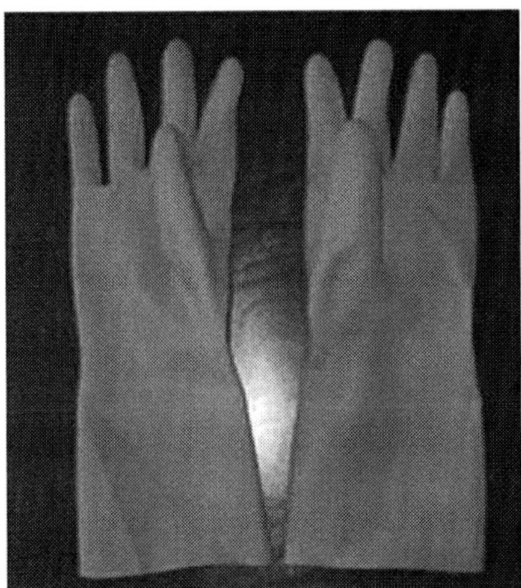

Fig. 9.1: Heavy duty gloves

Aprons, Gowns, Suits or Other Apparels

Aprons/gowns/suits are worn to prevent contamination of inner clothes and protect skin. It could be made either of cloth or impermeable material like plastic. People who work in incinerator chambers should wear gowns or suits made of non-inflammable material.

Masks/Eye Wear/Face Shields

A variety of masks (Fig. 9.2), eyewear, and face shields provide a protective barrier. It is compulsory for personnel working in the incinerator chamber to wear a mask covering both nose and mouth. A gas mask with filters is preferable.

Boots/Shoes

When splashes or large quantities of infected waste have to be handled, leg coverings, boots (Fig. 9.3) or shoe-covers provide greater protection to the skin. The boots should have rubber-sole and antiskidding property. They should cover the leg till the ankle.[9]

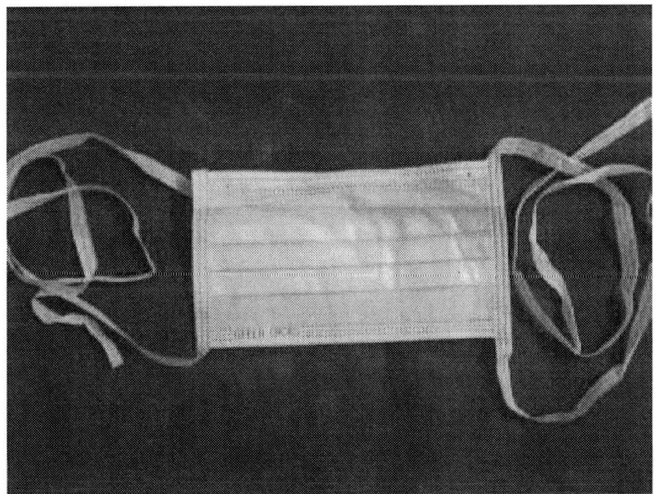

Fig. 9.2: Face mask

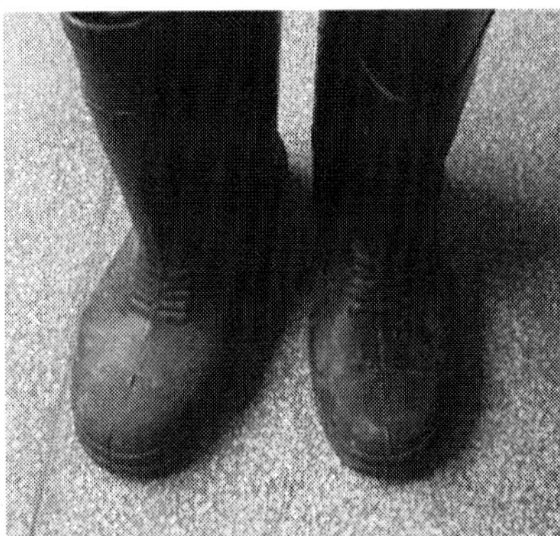

Fig. 9.3: Boots

Biomedical waste handling and transportation has three components:

1. Collection of different types of wastes from waste storage bags and containers inside the healthcare establishment.
2. On-site transportation and intermediate storage of segregated waste.
3. Off-site transportation of the waste towards the treatment or final disposal site.[8]

COLLECTION

To prevent accumulation of waste at the point of generation, the waste management plan should focus on establishing a routine for the collection of waste. Handling and transportation of waste containers should be done in such a manner that unnecessary exposure to staff and others is prevented. Transportation routes through the facility should be planned to minimize the movement of loaded waste carriers through patient care and other clean areas.[78]

- Avoid contaminating exterior surface of waste container. If this is not possible, ensure that external surface is decontaminated
- Avoid transportation of untreated waste through nonlab or high traffic corridors
- For transportation of liquid waste, secondary containers must be used which should be decontaminated after use

- Whenever possible, carts with raised sides should be used for transport.[62]

A strict protocol for collection of wastes should be adhered to by the auxiliary workers in charge of waste collection. It is the duty of the nursing and other clinical staff to ensure that waste bags are tightly closed or taped shut when they are three-quarters full. Light-gauge bags can be closed by tying the neck and heavier-gauge bags by self-locking plastic tags. Bags should never be stapled.

It should be strongly recommended that:

- Waste should be collected either on a daily basis or as frequently as required and transported to the designated central storage site
- Bags should be removed only after labeling with their respective sources of production (e.g. hospital, ward or department) and contents
- Ensure that the waste containers are immediately replaced with new ones when they are not more than three-quarters full
- Ensure that nonhazardous and hazardous/infectious health care wastes are collected on separate trolleys. The trolleys should also be marked with the corresponding color and washed regularly
- Empty collection bags/containers should be readily available at the point of waste generation[66]
- Waste collectors should be provided with heavy duty gloves, industrial boots and aprons.[9]

Procedure for Waste Collection

- Color-coded plastic bag should be kept in its container
- Biohazard symbol should be clearly displayed over the bags and containers
- As soon as it is 3/4th full of waste it should be removed from the container
- An infectious waste should never be mixed with the non-infectious waste
- Disposable items (syringes, catheters, IV bottles, rubber gloves, etc. should be collected after their chemical disinfection

and mutilation (by dipping in 1% hypochlorite solution for 30 min)

- Sharps should be kept in puncture proof labeled containers. Needles destroyer should be used to destroy needles. Other sharps waste should be chemically disinfected, mutilated/ shredded and then sent for final disposal
- Biomedical waste handlers should be trained in the proper waste handling procedures to avoid injury and accidents.[83]

STORAGE

Definition

Storage of biomedical waste means "the holding of biomedical waste for such period of time, at the end of which waste is treated and disposed off."[101]

A storage area for healthcare waste should be designated inside the healthcare or research facility and the biohazard symbol should be displayed. This area must be totally enclosed and separate from supply rooms and food preparation areas. The bags or containers, containing wastes should be stored in this separate area, room, or building of suitable size proportional to the quantity of waste produced and the frequency of collection.[66] Materials other than biomedical waste should never be placed in this storage area.

Floors, walls and ceilings of storage areas must be thoroughly cleaned according to the established guidelines of the facility, which are prepared in consultation with the facility's infection control committee, biosafety officer or other designated authority.[78] As per rules, biomedical waste can not be stored for more than 24 to 48 hours. However, if the storage room is refrigerated, wastes can be stored in bulk for over 48 hours.[83]

Recommendations for the storage area and its equipment are as follows:

- The storage area should have an impermeable, hard-standing floor with good drainage
- It should be easy to clean and disinfect
- It should be equipped with a water supply for cleaning purposes

- It should be easily accessible to the staff in charge of waste handling
- It should be provided with a lock to prevent access by un-authorized individuals
- It should provide an easy access to waste-collection vehicles
- It should be protected from the direct sunlight
- It must be inaccessible to animals, insects, and birds
- It should be well-illuminated and should afford passive ventilation
- It should not be situated near fresh food stores or food preparation areas such as canteens
- A supply of cleaning equipment, protective clothing, and waste bags or containers should be readily available to the storage area[66]
- It should be ideally situated on the ground floor near the rear entrance to make the transportation of waste to the site of final disposal easier
- It should have sufficient storage capacity for storing the required number of waste bags depending upon the quantity of waste generated in the hospital. It should be able to store waste generated in a minimum of two days
- To receive and dispatch the waste and to maintain proper record, a full time storekeeper should be there.[83]

If a refrigerated storage room is not available, storage times for healthcare waste should not exceed the following recommended duration:

In temperate climate:	72 hr in winter
	48 hr in summer
In warm climate:	48 hr during the winter
	24 hr during the summer[66]

Anatomical waste and all other infectious waste must be refrigerated at a temperature of 3 to 8°C, if stored for more than a week. The duration of storage for refrigerated or frozen biomedical and healthcare waste varies according to storage capacity, rate of waste generation and any other applicable local regulatory requirements.

Caution

- Infected glass or plastic items may fracture at lower temperatures
- Untreated infectious waste or waste with a high content of blood or other body fluids destined for off-site disposal (for which there is a risk of spilling) should never be compacted to decrease its volume
- Cytotoxic waste should be kept in a specific secure location separate from other healthcare waste
- Radioactive waste should be stored in lead containers to prevent dispersion. Waste that is to be stored till its radioactivity decay completes, should be labeled with the type of radionuclide, date, and detailed data of required storage conditions.[78]

TRANSPORTATION OF BIOMEDICAL WASTE

It means "movement of biomedical waste from the point of generation or collection to the final disposal".[101]

On-Site Transport

Healthcare waste needs to be transported within the healthcare establishment. This should be done by means of wheeled trolleys, containers, or carts (Fig. 9.4). These vehicles should be used for this purpose only and should not be used for any other purpose. The waste bags/containers should be placed securely in the trolley or cart.

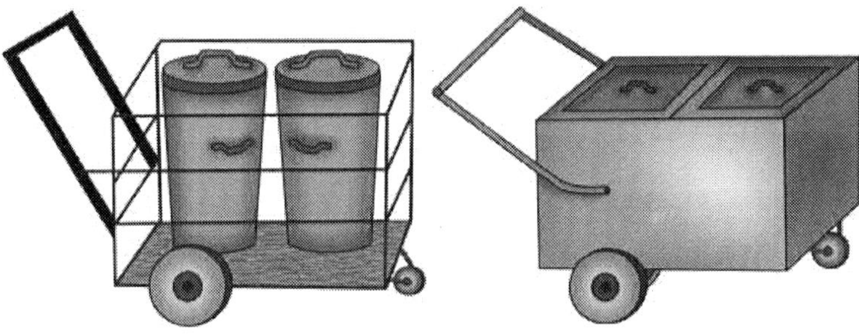

Fig. 9.4: Different types of on-site transportation vehicles (*Courtesy: WHO; Safe Management of Wastes from Healthcare Activities*)

These should meet the following specifications:

- Easy to load and unload
- No sharp edges that could damage waste bags or containers during loading and unloading
- Easy to clean.[66]

Transportation of waste should be done in compliance with the biomedical waste management rules. Waste handlers must be provided with uniform and personal protective equipment, i.e. apron, boots, gloves and masks, and these should always be worn while transporting the waste.[53]

Carts used for transporting healthcare waste through the healthcare facility should be designed to prevent spills, and should be made of materials which can withstand exposure to common cleaning agents. The biohazard symbol should be clearly displayed on carts used for the transport of infectious waste. All waste bag seals should be in place and intact at the end of transportation.

The vehicles should be cleaned and disinfected daily with an appropriate disinfectant. Alternatively, the frequency of cleaning and the type of cleaning agent to be used can be determined by consultation with the facility's infection control committee, biosafety officer or any other designated authority. Make sure that these carts are thoroughly cleaned before performing any maintenance work on them.[78]

It is recommended to use two sets of bins. It ensures proper collection of waste while the filled bins are being transported. These bins should also be cleaned/disinfected daily.[46]

Off-Site Transportation

Regulation and Control System

Off-site transportation is required when hazardous healthcare waste is treated outside the healthcare establishment. This requires that the healthcare waste must be labeled, displaying its nature and source. This is the responsibility of the waste producer to take care of proper packaging and labeling of the containers that are transported, and also for authorization of its destination. The logic behind labeling of healthcare waste bags/containers is that in case of an accident, the content can be easily identified and appropriate measures can be taken quickly.[91]

Packaging and labeling should be in compliance with national regulations governing the transport of hazardous wastes and with international agreements if wastes are to be shipped abroad for treatment.

The control strategy for transport of healthcare waste should include the following points:

- A consignment note for transportation of the waste should be handed over to the transporter at place of generation. On reaching the site of final disposal, the transporter should complete his part of the consignment note and return it to the waste producer.
- The transporting organization must be registered with the waste regulation authority.
- Handling and disposal facilities must hold a permit, issued by a waste regulation authority, which allows them to handle and dispose of healthcare waste.

Special Packaging Requirements for Off-Site Transport

The packaging should include the following essential elements:

Inner Packaging

It should comprise of:

- Waterproof primary container, made of metal or plastic with impermeable seal (e.g. a heat seal, a skirted stopper, or a metal crimp seal)
- A waterproof secondary packaging; if necessary to prevent perforations. Put a double bag if the exterior of the bag is contaminated
- Absorbent material placed between the primary receptacle and the secondary packaging to absorb the entire contents if accidental spillage occurs[66]
- Secondary containment should also be labeled with the biohazard symbol.[62]

Outer Packaging

It should be of adequate strength pertaining to its capacity, mass, and intended use. It should measure 100 mm in dimensions (minimum) on its exterior.

It is recommended to enclose a list of contents between the secondary packaging and the outer packaging. The outer packaging should be appropriately labeled.

The bags or containers should be sufficiently robust for their intended use (e.g. puncture-proof for sharps or resistant to aggressive chemicals) and for normal conditions of handling and transportation such as vibration or temperature changes, low or high relative humidity, or atmospheric pressure changes.

For infectious healthcare wastes, it is recommended that packaging should be design type—tested and certified as approved for use.

Packaging can be done in Two Possible Ways

- Rigid and leak-proof packaging [in compliance with a number of requirements and tests specified by the United Nations (1997)]
- Intermediate to large, rigid or flexible bulk containers, made from a variety of materials such as wood, plastics or textile [complying with a number of requirements and tests specified by the United Nations (1997)].

Packaging of intermediate bulk containers intended to contain sharp objects (e.g. broken glass and needles) should be puncture-resistant and shall undergo additional performance tests.

Vehicle design for off-site transportation of hazardous health-care waste (Fig. 9.5):

1. The body of the vehicle should be of appropriate size, with an internal body height of 2.2 meters.
2. The driver's cabin and the body (which is designed to retain the load) should be separate.

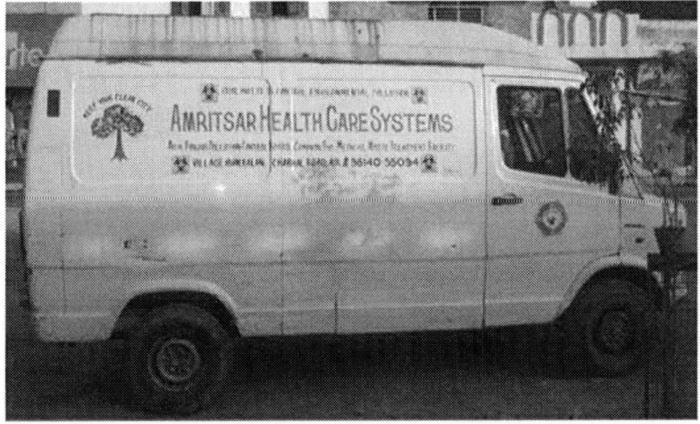

Fig. 9.5: Transportation vehicle
(*Courtesy*: Amritsar Enviro Care System (P) Ltd)
(Formerly Amritsar Healthcare Systems)

3. The load must be securely held in the vehicle during transport.
4. A separate compartment on the vehicle should contain empty plastic bags, suitable protective clothing, cleaning equipment, tools and disinfectant and special kits for dealing with liquid spills.
5. The internal finish of the vehicle should allow it to be steam-cleaned.
6. The internal corners should be rounded.
7. Name and address of the waste carrier must be displayed on the vehicle.
8. The international biohazard symbol and an emergency telephone number must be displayed on the vehicle or container.
9. For transporting hazardous healthcare waste, covered vehicles should be used.
10. Vehicles or containers dedicated for the transportation of hazardous healthcare waste should not be used for any other purpose. They should be sealed and kept locked at all times, except at the time of loading and unloading.
11. Articulated or demountable trailers (temperature controlled if required) are very useful for healthcare waste, as they can easily be left at the location of waste production.
12. Large containers can be used storage for storage as well as transportation of healthcare waste if dedicated vehicle is not available.

Routing

Healthcare waste should be transported by the quickest possible planned route. There should be no en route handling of waste. If handling is unavoidable, it should be prearranged and should take place in adequately designed and authorized premises. Handling requirements can have a specific mention in the contract signed between the waste generator and the carrier.[66]

Management of Accidents and Spillages

Spillage of infectious or other hazardous material or waste is probably the most common type of emergency in healthcare establishments. Response procedures are essentially the same regardless of whether the spillage involves waste or material in use:

- Contaminated areas should be cleaned (and disinfected, if required)
- Exposure of workers should be limited to the minimum during the clearing up operation
- The impact on patients, healthcare workers and the environment should be limited to the minimum.

One person should be designated with the responsibility of handling of emergencies, including coordination of actions, reporting to managers and regulators. Staff should be trained for expedited emergency response and the necessary equipment should be readily available at all times for safe and rapid implementation. Written procedures for the different kinds of emergencies should be drafted.

Most of the spillages are noninfectious and usually require only cleaning-up of the contaminated area. However for spillages of infectious material, it is important to ascertain the type of infectious agent (as in some cases, immediate evacuation of the area may be necessary). Usually more hazardous spillages occur in laboratories rather than in departments of the healthcare establishment.

Special Provisions for Needle Stick Injuries

Needles are one of the most dangerous items that are handled in a healthcare establishment due to their high potential for injuries and contamination. It is recommended to immediately disinfect the cuts inflicted by sharps.

Each healthcare establishment should put in place an accident reporting system. Any accident should be reported to the infection control nurse who will report this information to the competent authorities at central level.

It is highly recommended to perform postexposure blood investigations so as to after such an injury to ensure that the person has not been contaminated by any pathogen, particularly hepatitis B and C or HIV.

General Procedures to be Followed in Case of Spillages

1. Evacuate the contaminated area.
2. Decontaminate the eyes and skin of exposed personnel immediately and provide medical care and first aid.
3. Inform the designated authority who should coordinate the necessary actions.
4. Determine the nature of the spill and limit its spread.
5. Provide adequate Personal Protective Equipment (PPE) to personnel involved in cleaning up.
6. If indicated, neutralize or disinfect the spilled or contaminated material.
7. Collect all spilled and contaminated material and place this spilled material and disposable contaminated items used for its cleaning in the appropriate waste bags or containers.
8. Never pick up sharps by hand as it may cause injury. Instead, brushes, pans, etc. are recommended.
9. Disinfect or decontaminate the area and wipe up with absorbent cloth. Make sure that cloth or other absorbent material is never turned during this process as this spreads the contamination. The decontamination process should be started from the least contaminated area and terminated at the most contaminated area. The absorbent cloth must be changed at each stage of cleaning up. Dry cloths are recommended in case of liquid spillage; and cloth impregnated with appropriate water, i.e. acidic, basic, or neutral should be used for solid spills.
10. Thoroughly rinse the area and then wipe dry with absorbent cloths.
11. Decontaminate or disinfect all the used tools.
12. Remove PPE and decontaminate/disinfect it if required, as in case of reusable apparel.
13. Seek immediate medical attention if exposure to hazardous material has occurred during the procedure of clean up.[91]

CHAPTER

10 Treatment and Disposal

WASTE TREATMENT

Here the term 'treatment' refers to the process of modifying the waste in some way before it is taken to its final resting place. Treatment is required to decontaminate or disinfect the waste at source so that it no longer acts as the source of pathogenic organisms. After such treatment, the residual matter can be safely handled, transported and stored.[40]

The choice of treatment method should be decided according to:

a. The type, nature and volume of the wastes.
b. The hazard and viability of the pathogenic organisms in the waste.
c. The efficiency of the treatment method.
d. The conditions at which the treatment method operates.
e. The cost-effectiveness of the treatment method.[78]

Why do we Need Treatment of Hospital Waste?

Treatment of waste is required:

- To disinfect the waste so that it no longer acts as the source of infection
- To reduce the volume of the waste needing disposal
- To make waste unrecognizable to public for esthetic reasons
- To make recycled items unusable.[20]

Biomedical waste shall be treated and disposed off in accordance with Schedule I, and in compliance with the standards prescribed in Schedule V (of Biomedical Waste Management Rules, 1998). Every occupier, where required, shall set up in accordance with the time schedule in schedule VI requisite biomedical waste treatment facilities like incinerator, autoclave, microwave system for the treatment of waste or, ensure requisite treatment of waste at a Common Waste Treatment Facility (CWTF) or any other waste treatment facility.[51]

Wherever possible, healthcare establishments should use nearby CWTF. They should sign a contract with such CWTFs for the collection, treatment and disposal of the biomedical waste. If access to a CWTF is difficult, the healthcare establishments should manage the potentially infected biomedical waste as given below:[53]

Hazardous/infectious healthcare waste can be treated to reach an acceptable level of hazard/infectiousness. This allows these wastes to follow the nonrisk healthcare waste stream and their disposal with the general solid waste. Alternatively, they can be directly disposed of in sanitary landfills or by incineration. Minimal observances for waste treatment and disposal:

As per National Healthcare Waste Management (NHCWM) plan, it is a legal binding to ensure that:

- The most hazardous healthcare waste (i.e. sharps) and highly infectious waste are properly treated and disposed off in healthcare establishments all over the country
- Treatment/disposal options recommended in the NHCWM plan are homogeneously applied in the country
- The selected options are compatible with the local capacities of operation and maintenance
- Most environment friendly and cost-effective options are selected.

Hazardous/infectious healthcare waste can either be treated on-site, i.e. in the healthcare facility itself, or off-site, i.e. in another healthcare facility or in a dedicated treatment plant (CWTF). Table 10.1 gives merits and demerits of both treatment facilities.[91]

Guidelines for Biomedical Waste Management Facilities

1. Biomedical waste segregation, collection, storage, treatment and disposal must be practiced or outsourced according to Biomedical Waste Management Rules.
2. In designing the layout of a facility, movement of waste should be properly planned.

Table 10.1: Advantages and disadvantages of on-site and off-site treatment facilities

Sr. No.	*On-site*	*Off-site*
1.	It is the only a possible option in rural healthcare establishments of primary sector.	It is a better option when a number of healthcare establishments are in vicinity of the CWTF.
2.	Can also be carried out in major rural healthcare establishments where huge amounts of health-care waste is generated.	It is carried out on the outskirts of a city and collects waste from more than one healthcare establishment.
3.	Poor road and transport system is not a hurdle.	It is a major hurdle for transportation of waste from one place to other.
4.	It is more convenient and ensures direct supervision by the occupier.	Transportation of waste is inconvenient.
5.	Risks to public health and environment is minimized because hazardous/infection healthcare waste remains confined to the healthcare establishment.	It always carries this risk while transportation.
6.	Treatment costs are high because of high cost of monitoring and surveillance as well as flue-gas cleaning.	Relatively cost-effective as these costs are reduced.
7.	Extra technical staff is required for operation and maintenance of facilities.	Skilled workers are readily available who operate and maintain the CWTF effectively.
8.	Supervision and monitoring of many small facilities by relevant govt. agencies is difficult. bags, etc. can be reduced.	It is easy to supervise and monitor a CWTF and malpractices such as reuse of needles, syringes, blood
9.	Show poor compliance with operating standards.	Compliance with operating standard is better.
10.	Environment pollution cannot be kept under check in an effective way.	Environment pollution can be kept under check in an effective way.
11.	Healthcare establishment will have to devote time and personnel to manage their own installations.	No such problems.
12.	Future modifications or expansions to match the changing standards and limits in relation to emission of pollutants will be a costly fair.	These modification will be less expensive.
13.	Privatization, if planned in future, will be difficult to achieve in many small units.	It will be easier on regional basis.

Source: *United Nations Environment Program/SBC*

3. Appropriate storage bins and collection equipment for various categories of biomedical waste should be provided.
4. Lockable storage area temporary storage of segregated infectious waste should be provided where waste can be kept prior to disposal or transport to other facilities for disposal.
5. If there is not any access to CWTF, areas for sharps pit and deep burial pits should be earmarked.[53]

Centralized Facility for Biomedical Waste Management

Centralized waste management facilities are run by private waste companies. State branch of IMA (Indian Medical Association), on behalf of healthcare establishments, and in collaboration with state pollution control board, find a private operator of centralized waste treatment facility. State Pollution Control Board conducts a tender bid and a private operator is identified. Then IMA and operator chalk out a mutually acceptable cost of disposal which is calculated on per-bed or per-kg basis.

It must be noted that even though a CWTF will take care of final disposal, it is the duty of healthcare establishments to ensure proper segregation and treatment before collection and transportation of waste to the facility.[23]

Disinfection

It is a process of destruction or removal of pathogens which give rise to infection. Disinfection should be used despite of sterilization facilities. Infectious waste should be disinfected before its disposal. Instruments and equipments that come in contact with infected waste, contaminated floor, clothes, bedding, beds, surfaces like trolley tops, table tops and utensils, etc. should be regularly disinfected.[44]

The relative effectiveness of treatment methods depends on numerous factors including:

1. *Pathological organisms*: The volume, concentration, type and viability of the organism in the waste.
2. *Material to be disinfected*: Its physiological state and diffusion resistance.
3. *Treatment method:* Operating parameters and conditions.

These methods of treatment can be used in combination also so that waste can be inactivated and safely discharged. The choice is determined on the basis of risk assessment requirements and/or discharge consent standards.[78]

CATEGORY-WISE MANAGEMENT OF BIOMEDICAL WASTE

A category-wise management of biomedical waste is given below:

Human Anatomical Waste and Animal Waste (Category 1 and 2)

Keeping in view the public sensitivity, waste human body parts, organs and tissues must be handled with extra care.[38] The waste must be collected in yellow bags as soon as possible at the source only.[91] Human anatomical waste and most animal waste, consisting of human/animal tissues, organs, and body parts, carcasses, bedding, fluid blood and blood products, items saturated or dripping with blood, body fluids contaminated with blood, and body fluids removed for diagnosis or removed during surgery, treatment or autopsy must be incinerated in a biomedical waste incinerator.

Microbiological and Biotechnological Waste (Category 3)

Highly infectious waste, such as lab cultures, stocks of infectious agents from laboratory work, human or animal cell cultures used in research must be incinerated, autoclaved or chemically disinfected.[38]

Waste Sharps (Category 4)

Sharps are anything that may cause puncture or cuts and include needles, scalpels, blades, broken glass, syringes, slides, lancets, suture needles, and IV catheters. The safe disposal of used or unused sharps is a critical component of a biomedical waste management program.

- Sharps should never be left casually on counter tops, food trays, beds as grave injuries can occur

- Segregation and storage of sharps must be done in puncture-proof containers at the point of generation only.

Treatment of sharps is done according to following sequence:

DISINFECTION → MUTILATION
→ SECURED LANDFILL
→ SHARPS PIT
→ ENCAPSULATION[53]

Disinfection

Disinfection of sharps is achieved by:

- Treatment with 1 percent hypochlorite solution or any other equivalent chemical reagent.
- Autoclaving/microwaving/hydroclaving.

Mutilation

Material Reprocessing

a. *Plastic reprocessing*: After treatment, the shredded plastic from syringes is sent for material recovery by the formal or informal sector. The hospitals should ensure that disinfected and mutilated waste is sent for material recovery so that the safety of people working in the material recovery industry is not compromised.

b. *Metal reprocessing*: Reprocessing of the sharps is considered a better alternative to the present methods of sharps management. Smelting of metals is considered as one of the final disposal options.[100]

Even syringes without needles should be considered as unsafe. Used syringes, needles or safety boxes should neither be disposed of in regular garbage nor be dumped randomly without prior treatment.

Disposal of Syringe along with Needle

The whole combination of "syringe plus needle" is dropped into a safety box immediately after use, which is then treated with other infectious waste. The idea is to reduce the risk of needle-stick injuries to the medical staff. It generates sharp waste in larger amount. Incineration at temperatures above 1400°C can oxidize the needles completely which is possible to achieve in pyrolytic incinerators or rotary kilns. Alternatively, air-excess incinerators or improved double-chamber autocombustion incinerators can be used. These operate at temperatures of 800 to 900°C and can burn the syringes and disinfect the needles. However the problem with this process is that ash still contains the needles, and hence must be carefully handled during burial.

Separate Disposal of Needle and Syringe

It enables to reduce the volume of infectious sharps waste by more than 90 percent. Needles are separated from the syringes and are isolated in a puncture-proof container and then disposed off by burning, incineration, or burial.

There are three ways separate the needle from the syringe, i.e. needle remover, needle cutter or needle destroyer.

Needle Remover

Needle is inserted into a slot of a container which is specially designed to separate it from the syringe using one hand only. The needle drops in the container made of polyethylene (closed tube or empty drug-boxes, cans, etc.). Once full, the container is safely emptied into a sharp pit and encapsulated.

Needle Cutters

These devices are installed at the site of use for cutting the needle from the syringe immediately after use. The needle is inserted into the device, and cut off mechanically with the help of blades. The needle drops into a container, which once full, can either be emptied in a sharp pit or incinerated. They are relatively cheap, safe, robust, easy to use and transport, and appropriate in remote areas where electricity supply may be lacking.

Needle Destroyers (Fig. 10.1)

These are relatively expensive devices, in which the needle is destroyed at the point of using an electrical current. The needle is inserted into a hole or slot in the device, which guides and positions the needle between two electrodes in the interior of the device. By simultaneous contact of needle with both electrodes,

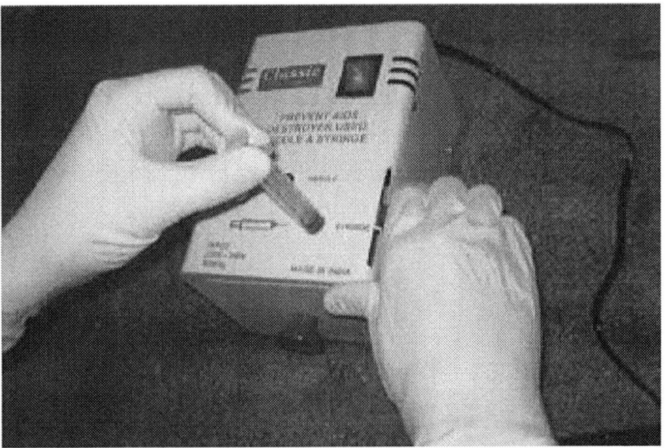

Fig. 10.1: Needle destroyer cum needle cutter

electric current runs through the needle which heats it to temperatures in the range of 1500 to 3000°C. This results in a partial or total oxidation of the needle.[91]

Final Disposal

As per rules, after disinfection and mutilation, sharps should be disposed in secured landfills as per the rules. As secured landfills are not available everywhere, the following alternate systems are recommended.

Sharps Pit (Fig. 10.2)

As per the guidelines of Biomedical Waste (Management and Handling) Rules, 1998, sharps pit should have following essential features.

The pit can be circular or rectangular in shape, which can be dug and lined with brick, masonry or concrete rings. The pit must be covered with a heavy concrete slab. The slab should be which is penetrated by a galvanized steel pipe projecting about 1.5 m above the slab, with an internal diameter of up to 20 mm. Once the pit is full, it can be sealed completely.

Note: A new pit should be ready before the pit in-use is full.

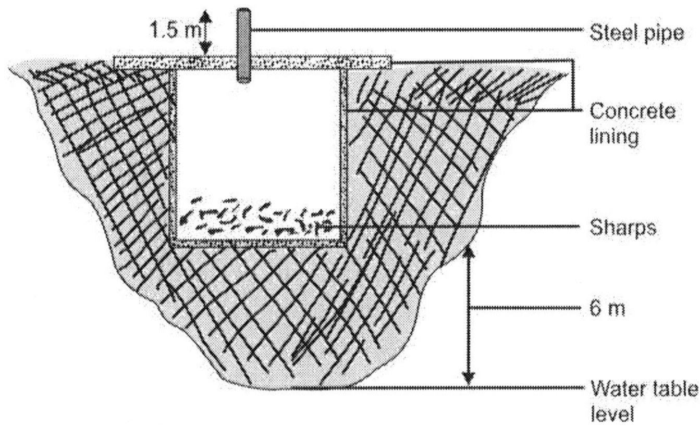

Fig. 10.2: Sharps pit

Encapsulation (Fig. 10.3)

As per WHO (1999) recommendations, encapsulation is the easiest method for the safe disposal of sharps. The puncture-proof and leak-proof containers are used for collection of sharps. When a container is three-quarter full, a material such as cement mortar, epoxy, grout, bitumen, clay or plastic foam is poured into fill the container completely. After the medium has dried, the containers are sealed and disposed off in landfill sites.[100]

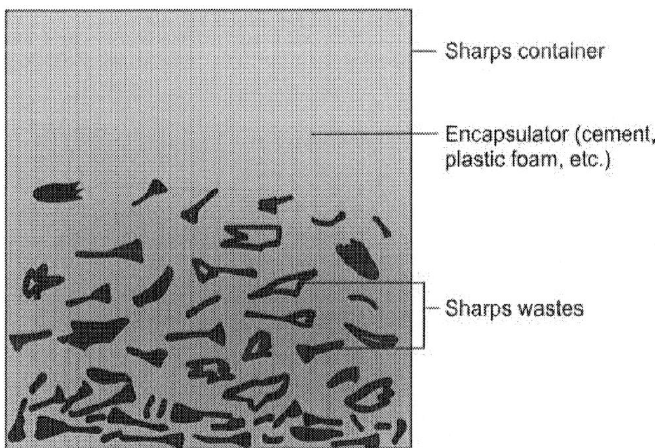

Fig. 10.3: Encapsulation

The encapsulation of sharps wastes for ultimate disposal in a waste disposal ground should follow certain criteria, regardless of the encapsulating material used. These are:

1. The encapsulating mixture must be fluid enough to penetrate the collected sharps to the bottom of the container.
2. The encapsulating mixture must completely surround all the collected sharps wastes.
3. The encapsulating mixture must set to form a rigid mass before disposal in a waste disposal ground.
4. The encapsulator must not show expansion; else it will burst the sharps wastes container.

Encapsulation ensures that individual sharps are not freed through an inadvertent bursting of the sharps wastes container even during compaction of waste material using heavy equipment (which is sometimes used to reduce the volume of the waste on waste disposal grounds).

Advantages

1. It is an effective method of sharps disposal in areas where neither a biomedical waste treatment facility nor a dedicated biomedical waste area at a waste disposal ground is available.
2. Encapsulated sharps wastes can be discarded in the general waste at the generator's healthcare establishments.
3. The materials used for encapsulation are easily available everywhere and are not so expensive.
4. The procedure is simple to understand and execute.[54]

Discarded Medicine and Cytotoxic Drugs (Category 5)

Whereas disposal of small quantity of chemical or pharmaceutical waste is easy and relatively cheap, large amounts require the use of special treatment facilities.

Disposal of Small Quantities of Pharmaceutical Waste

The following are the disposal options for small quantities of pharmaceutical waste:

1. *Disposal to a landfill*: Pharmaceutical waste produced in small quantity on a daily basis may be landfilled. However, it should be dispersed in large quantity of general waste.

   Note: Cytotoxic and narcotic drugs should never be landfilled, even in small quantity.
2. *Encapsulation*: Small quantities of pharmaceutical waste may be appropriately encapsulated, along with sharps.
3. *On-site safe burial*: On-site safe burial of small amount of pharmaceutical waste prevents scavenging. It may be an appropriate disposal method for establishments applying minimal programs for biomedical waste disposal.
4. *Discharge to a sewer*: Relatively mild liquid or semiliquid pharmaceuticals, such as solutions containing vitamins, cough syrups, intravenous solutions, eyedrops, etc. in moderate quantity can be discharged into municipal sewer. These should be diluted in a large flow of water and then discharged into municipal sewers. But antibiotics and cytotoxic drugs should never be discharged into sewer. Also discharge of even small quantity of pharmaceutical waste into slow-moving or stagnant water bodies is unacceptable.
5. *Incineration*: Pharmaceutical wastes release toxic emission to the air if incinerated. However, small quantity of pharmaceutical waste may be incinerated together with infectious or general waste, provided it does not form greater than 1 percent of the total waste.
6. *Inertization*: This process involves mixing waste with cement and other substances before disposal so as to minimize the risk of migration of toxic substances contained in the waste into surface water or groundwater. This process is particularly suitable for pharmaceuticals and for incineration ashes with a high metal content. In the latter case, the process is also called as 'stabilization'.

For the inertization of pharmaceutical waste, its packaging should be removed and the pharmaceuticals should be ground. Then a mixture of water, lime and cement is added to the ground pharmaceutical waste to yield a homogeneous mass. Cubes or pellets of this mixture are formed on site which can be transported to a suitable storage site. As an alternative, the homogeneous mixture can be transported in liquid state only to a landfill and then poured into municipal waste.

The typical proportions for the mixture are:
Pharmaceutical waste—65 percent
Lime—15 percent
Cement—5 percent
Water—5 percent.

Advantages

- Inertization is reasonably inexpensive
- It is a simple process and can be performed using relatively unsophisticated equipment
- The main requirements are operating personnel, a grinder or road roller to grind the pharmaceuticals, a concrete mixer, and supplies of cement, lime, and water.

Disposal of Large Quantities of Pharmaceutical Waste

Large quantities of solid pharmaceutical waste are produce if a pharmacy closes down or after emergencies. The possible methods for disposal of such huge amounts of pharmaceutical waste are given below.

Incineration

Incineration is the best way for disposal of pharmaceutical waste. To ensure optimal combustion conditions, these wastes should be mixed with their cardboard packaging, and possibly with other combustible material and infectious waste. As low-temperature incineration (<800°C), provides only partial treatment for this type of waste, it must be followed by combustion in a second chamber, operating at temperatures about 1000°C, to burn off potentially toxic exhaust gases. Incinerators designed for industrial waste (including rotary kilns), which can operate at high temperatures (>1200°C) are ideal for large amounts of pharmaceuticals. Cement kilns can also be used, provided that pharmaceutical material does not exceed 5 percent of the fuel fed into the furnace at any time.

Encapsulation

Landfilling of large quantities of pharmaceuticals is not recommended unless the waste is encapsulated. So solid, liquid, and semiliquid waste should be encapsulated in metal drums prior to landfilling as there is risk of groundwater contamination is minimized. Large amounts of pharmaceutical waste should neither be disposed of with general hospital waste, nor be diluted and discharged into sewers. However, certain very mild solutions, such as vitamin preparations can be discharged down the drain. Intravenous fluids such as glucose, salts, amino acids, lipids, etc. can be disposed off to a landfill or discharged into a sewer as these are relatively harmless.

Ampoules should be crushed on a hard, impermeable surface. During this procedure, workers should wear necessary personal protective equipment. The crushed glass should then be swept up, collected, and disposed off with sharps. Ampoules should never be incinerated as they may explode and cause damage to the incinerator or injury to the workers.

Cytotoxic Waste

As cytotoxic waste is highly hazardous, it should never be landfilled or discharged into the sanitary sewer. Disposal options include:

1. *Return to original supplier*

The manufacturers should run a 'take back' policy for such drugs because the manufacturer has the infrastructure to handle these drugs. Outdated drugs and drugs that are no longer required but safely packaged should be returned to the supplier. This is the preferred option for countries that lack the facilities for incineration.

Drugs that have been unpacked should be repackaged in similar manner like original packaging and marked as "outdated" or "not for use".

2. *Incineration at high temperatures (Table 10.2)*

Complete destruction of all cytotoxic substances may require temperatures up to 1200°C. Incineration at lower temperatures may result in partial combustion leading to the release of hazardous cytotoxic vapors into the atmosphere. Modern double-chamber pyrolytic incinerators can be used as they can operate at tempera-

Table 10.2: Minimum temperatures for destruction of cytotoxic drugs for conventional residence times

Compound	*Temperature*	*Compound*	*Temperature*
Aclarubicin	1000°C	Cyclophosphamide	900°C
Bleomycin	1000°C	Etoposide	1000°C, 700°C
Carboplatin	1000°C	5-Fluorouracil	1200°C, 1000°C, 700°
Cisplatin	250°C, 500°C	Melphalan	500°C
Methotrexate	1000°C	Mitomycin	1000°C
Vincristine	1000°C	Doxorubicin	700°C

Source: *Pruss A, Giroult E, Rushbrook, Safe Management of Waste from Healthcare Activities (WHO).*

ture of 1200°C, with a minimum gas residence time of 2 seconds or 1000°C with a minimum gas residence time of 5 seconds in the second chamber.

Incineration can also be carried out in:

a. Rotary kilns designed for thermal decomposition of chemical wastes
b. Foundries or
c. Cement kilns which usually have furnaces operating well in excess of 850°C.

Incineration in most municipal incinerators, in single chamber incinerators, or by open-air burning is not appropriate for the disposal of cytotoxic waste.

Chemical Degradation

Chemical degradation methods for conversion of cytotoxic compounds into nontoxic/nongenotoxic compounds can be used for drug residues, cleaning of contaminated urinals, spillages, and protective clothing. Most of these methods are relatively simple and safe to use. The methods are:

1. Oxidation by potassium permanganate ($KMnO_4$) or sulfuric acid (H_2SO_4).
2. Denitrozation by hydrobromic acid (HBr).
3. Reduction by nickel and aluminum.

Note: Neither incineration nor chemical degradation currently provides a completely satisfactory solution for the treatment of waste, spillages or biological fluids contaminated by antineoplastic agents. So hospitals should use the utmost care in the use and handling of cytotoxic drugs. Encapsulation or inertization may be considered as a last resort for:

1. Areas where neither high-temperature incineration nor chemical degradation methods are available.
2. Countries where it is not possible to export the cytotoxic wastes for adequate treatment to a country with the necessary facilities and expertise.[66]

Table 10.3 summarizes the methods for disposal of various categories of pharmaceuticals.[24]

Soiled Waste (Category 6)

Human blood, blood products, body fluids contaminated with blood, and body fluids removed for diagnosis or removed during surgery, treatment or autopsy (except urine or feces) should be first disinfected by chemical decontamination or steam autoclave, and then these may be discharged down the sanitary sewer. It should be remembered that only those wastes which are not associated with exotic communicable diseases can be handled in this manner.

These fluids should be handled with extra care so as to prevent spills and the formation of aerosols. These fluids should never be disposed in the sewer if untreated.

Items saturated or dripping with blood, such as disposable surgical drapes, surgical gowns, sponges, dressings, etc. should be incinerated, autoclaved or chemically disinfected. However, reusable materials saturated with blood may be laundered or reprocessed and should not be considered waste.[38]

Solid Waste (Category 7)

Solid wastes including plastic waste are often infected. These are first disinfected and shredded at source so as to render them unusable. Ultimate disposal is by either recycling or municipal landfill.[51]

Liquid Waste (Category 8)

Liquid waste generated from laboratory washing, cleaning and disinfecting activities has to be disinfected by chemical treatment before discharging in drain. However, it is not practical to disinfect

Table 10.3: Disposal methods for pharmaceutical wastes

Category	*Disposal methods*	*Comments*
Solids Semisolids Powders	Landfill Waste encapsulation Waste inertization Medium and high temperature incineration (cement kiln incinerator)	No more than 1% of the daily municipal waste should be disposed of daily in an untreated form (non-immobilized) to a landfill.
Liquids	Sewer High temperature incineration (cement kiln incinerator)	Antineoplastics not to sewer.
Ampoules	Crush ampoules and flush diluted fluid to sewer	Antineoplastics not to sewer.
Anti-infective drugs	Waste encapsulation Waste inertization Medium and high temperature incineration (cement kiln incinerator)	Liquid antibiotics may be diluted with water, left to stand for several weeks and discharged to a sewer
Antineoplastic drugs	Return to donor or manufacturer Waste encapsulation Waste inertization Medium and high temperature incineration (cement kiln incinerator) (chemical decomposition)	Not to landfill unless encapsulated Not to sewer. No medium temperature incineration.
Paper, cardboard	Recycle, burn, landfill	
Controlled drugs	Waste encapsulation Waste inertization Medium and high temperature incineration (cement kiln incinerator)	Not to landfill unless encapsulated.
Aerosol canisters	Landfill Waste encapsulation	Not to be burnt: May explode.
Disinfectants	Use to sewer or fast-flowing watercourse: Small quantities of diluted disinfectants (max. 50 liters per day under supervision)	No undiluted disinfectants to sewers or water courses. Maximum 50 liters per day diluted to sewer or fast-flowing watercourse. No disinfectants at all to slow moving or stagnant watercourses.
PVC plastic, glass	Landfill	Not for burning in open containers.

Source: *Deliver, World Health Organization. Guidelines for the Storage of Essential Medicines and Other Health Commodities. Arlington.*

huge volumes of liquid waste. Instead, the practice of disinfection for blood containers is a better approach. Blood samples received for analysis are carefully decanted in metal kettles and are autoclaved in disposal autoclave. The small amount of residual blood in the containers is disinfected by hypochlorite. The routine washing procedures (after disinfection of the labware contaminated with blood or body fluids) could be discharged in the drain.[22]

Incineration Ash (Category 9)

Ash produced due to incineration of any biomedical waste is disposed off in municipal landfill or disposed off by inertization.[51]

Chemical Waste (Category 10)

Chemical waste needs special treatment and disposal. So efforts should be done to minimize the chemical waste.

Disposal of General Chemical Waste

General chemical waste which cannot be recycled such as sugars, amino acids and certain salts can be disposed of with general municipal waste or discharged into municipal sewers.

Petroleum spirit, calcium carbide, and halogenated organic solvents should not be discharged into sewers.

Disposal of Hazardous Chemical Waste

Small Quantity

Unauthorized discharge of hazardous chemicals into the sewer can be dangerous to sewage treatment workers. These hazardous chemicals may also adversely affect the functioning of sewage treatment works.

Hazardous chemical waste in small quantity, e.g. residual chemicals inside their packaging can be treated by encapsulation, landfilling or pyrolytic oxidation.

Large Quantities

Hazardous chemical waste in large quantity should not be discharged into sewer, buried or encapsulated. The nature of the hazard posed by the waste determines the appropriate means of disposal.

1. *Incineration*: Certain combustible wastes, may be incinerated, but large quantity of halogenated solvents should not be incinerated if facilities do not have adequate gas-cleaning equipment.
2. *Return to the original supplier*: Most of the times suppliers are better equipped to deal with them in a safe way. The facilities should include such provisions in the original purchase contract for the chemicals. If such provisions are not available in the home country, the waste could also be exported to a country having the expertise and facilities to deal with hazardous wastes.

Wastes Containing High Heavy Metals

Incineration of wastes containing mercury or cadmium is not recommended because toxic vapors produced during this process cause atmospheric pollution. Neither these should be disposed of in municipal landfills as they may leach out and pollute the groundwater. The treatment options are:

1. Recovery of heavy metals at specialized.
2. Return to the suppliers of the original equipment.
3. Disposal in a safe storage site designed specifically for the final disposal of hazardous industrial waste.
4. Encapsulation and subsequent disposal in an impermeable landfill.

Pressurized Containers

Pressurized containers or aerosol cans should never be incinerated because they may explode. Instead, they should be recycled/ reused or sent back to the gas suppliers for refilling.

Undamaged Containers

These should be returned to the supplier, e.g.

- Pressurized cylinders for oxygen, nitrogen, compressed air, carbon dioxide, cyclopropane, hydrogen, liquid petroleum gas and acetylene (for welding)
- Nitrous oxide cartridges or cylinders attached directly to the anesthesia equipment

- Ethylene oxide cartridges or cylinders attached to specially designed sterilizers.

Damaged Containers

1. Damaged pressurized containers which are not suitable for refilling: When it is uneconomical to return the empty containers to the gas suppliers, these should be emptied completely, crushed and then disposed of in any landfill.
2. The other option is recovery of metals at specified 'cottage' industries.
3. For containers having residual pressure but corroded valves, it is recommended and the only safe solution that they should be assembled, and destroyed by controlled explosion at a safe location by qualified specialists.

Radioactive Waste

Options for management of radioactive healthcare waste

1. Release from regulatory control immediately or after a period of decay storage (from days to a few years), as per the quantity or at activity levels established by the regulatory authority.
2. Return the waste to the producer/supplier of the original material, specially large sealed sources and sources containing long-lived radionuclides.
3. If none of these options is feasible, the waste can be sent to a disposal facility or a facility for long-term storage for future disposal. In both cases, prior treatment or conditioning of waste is required.

Recycling and Reuse

If circumstances permit, this option should be considered as an alternative to disposal. The possible options are:

- Reuse of sealed sources
- Decontamination and reuse of equipment and protective clothing
- Reuse of dilute waste streams for the purpose of rinsing and washing of waste tanks that contained liquid waste with higher radioactivity content.

Return to Supplier

The radioactive items may become waste if they possess damaged conditioning, decayed activity or if they are no longer required. Spent sources used for teletherapy also become waste.

Spent sealed sources with high activity and those containing long-lived radionuclides can also be returned to suppliers.

Hospitals may send nonrecyclable spent sealed sources to an authorized facility, a nuclear industry with appropriate capabilities or to the national agency designated for radioactive waste disposal. If any healthcare institution plans to import a sealed source containing radioactive material (having an activity >100 MBq), it is recommended that after 10 years of receipt, it should:

- Return the spent material to the supplier after expiry of its useful lifetime. This proposal should be included in the contract between the healthcare establishment and the supplier that the supplier would accept the radioactive waste within 1 year of such return being requested. Also that the user would return the source to the supplier not later than 15 years after receiving it.
- Submit a copy of relevant parts of the contract or acceptance document to the regulatory authority.

Treatment and Conditioning

Whenever necessary, treatment and conditioning of radioactive waste should be done so as to improve the characteristics of waste before interim storage and/or disposal. Treatment includes operations intended to change the characteristics of the radioactive waste and hence improve safety or economy. The basic objectives of treatment given in the Table 10.4.

Important

Treatment processes may result in the production of secondary radioactive waste streams such as contaminated filters, sludges, spent resins, ash, etc. which also require appropriate management.

Table 10.4: Various objectives and methods of disposal of radioactive wastes

S. No.	Objective	For solid waste	For liquid waste
1.	Removal of radionucleotides	Decontamination	Ion exchange
2.	Volume reduction	• Shredding • Low-force compaction Controlled incineration	Evaporation under controlled condition
3.	Change of composition	-------------	Precipitation Filtration

Source: *Safe Management of Waste from Healthcare Activities (WHO).*

Discharge/Disposal

The healthcare institution should ensure that radionuclides are released to the environment only when it is confirmed that:

- The activity of the released waste is below the clearance levels; or
- The activity of the discharged liquid or gaseous effluents is within limits authorized by the regulatory authority.

If a healthcare institution wishes to release solid, liquid, or gaseous radioactive waste with activity above the clearance levels to the environment, it should apply for an authorization to do so. It should also:

- Keep the radioactive discharge as far below the authorized limits as is reasonably achievable
- Monitor and keep a detailed and accurate record of the discharges or releases of radionuclides to demonstrate compliance with the authorized discharge limits
- Report discharges to the regulatory authority at specified intervals
- Report to the regulatory authority immediately if any discharges or releases that exceed the authorized limits
- When it is not suitable for a radioactive to be discharged or released to the environment or for cleared within a reasonable time, the healthcare institution should submit its proposals for disposal to the regulatory authority.

Management of Individual Radioactive Item

1. *Disposable syringes (used for radiotherapy)*: Empty them at a designated location → store in a sharps container till complete decay of residual activity occurs, if any → disposal of syringes and needles as normally done.
2. *Radioactive solid waste*: Do not disinfect solid radioactive waste by steam based, i.e. autoclave or microwave procedures. Solid radioactive waste, e.g. bottles, glassware, containers, etc. must be destroyed before disposal to avoid reuse by the public.
3. *Drainage system*: The drains designated for discharge of radioactive liquids should be identified. In case repairs become necessary, it is recommended to measure radiation levels as the drain or sewers is opened up, and take appropriate precautions.
4. *Liquids radioactive waste*: Interim storage of higher-level radioactive waste of relatively short half-life, (e.g. from iodine-131 therapy) and liquids that are immiscible with water (e.g. scintillation counting residues and contaminated oil) for decay in lead-shielded and marked container is recommended. These should be stored until activities reach the activity levels below the authorized clearance levels.

   Water-miscible waste may then be discharged to the sewer system and immiscible waste may be disposed of by the same methods as used for large quantities of hazardous chemical waste.
5. *Radioactive spills:* Radioactive waste resulting from cleaning-up operations after a spillage or other accident should be stored in suitable containers, until the activity reaches a level far below the permissible limits for discharge. However, waste with excessive activity accidently enters the sewer flow, a large volume of water to dilute the radioactivity to about 1 kBq per liter.
6. *Patient's excreta:* It is not usually necessary to collect and confine patient's excreta after diagnostic and therapeutic procedures. However, ordinary toilets used by such patients must be checked regularly for radioactive contamination by competent staff, (e.g. the Radiation Officer).

7. *Radioactive gases:* The radioactive gases generated during research and radioimmunoassays, should be discharged directly to the atmosphere for dilution by dispersal, but within the authorized limits. The site and design for exit of all gaseous waste discharges, including exhausts from stores and fume cupboards, should be such that it should prevent re-entry into any part of the premises.[66]

METHODS FOR TREATMENT OF BIOMEDICAL WASTE

The methods for treatment of waste can be classified as:

A. Incineration.
B. Nonincineration methods.[71]

Incineration

Definition

Incineration is a high temperature dry oxidation process, which reduces organic and combustible waste to inorganic incombustible matter.[83]

Incinerators operate at very high temperatures (1800°F and above) to combust waste products. All types of pathogens are completely destroyed at such high temperatures, and so incineration is very effective method of waste treatment.[72] This method is usually indicated for the waste that cannot be reused, recycled or disposed off in landfill site.

Characteristics of waste to be incinerated include:

a. Combustible matter above 60 percent in content.
b. Noncombustible matter below 50 percent in content.
c. Noncombustible fines below 20 percent in content.
d. Moisture content below 30 percent.
e. Low heating volume—above 2000 Kcal/kg for single chamber incinerators; above 3500 Kcal/kg for pyrolytic double chamber incinerators.

Waste types contraindicated for incineration are:

a. Halogenated plastics such as Polyvinyl Chloride (PVC).
b. Waste with high cadmium or mercury content, e.g. broken thermometers, used batteries.

c. Sealed ampoules or ampoules containing heavy metals.
d. Pressurized gas containers.
e. Large bulk of reactive chemical wastes.
f. Photographic or radiographic wastes and silver salts.

Types of Incinerators

1. *Double chamber pyrolytic incinerator (Fig. 10.4):* This is the most commonly used type of incinerators. In the first pyrolytic chamber, i.e. pyrolytic chamber, waste undergoes combustion in oxygen deficient conditions at 800°C. This results in production of solid ashes and gases. These gases are burnt in the second chamber at high temperature ranging from 900 to 1200°C, using an excess of air to minimize smoke and odor. This equipment is bit expensive and requires trained personnel to handle it.
2. *Single chamber furnaces with static grate:* These are indicated only if pyrolytic incinerators are unaffordable.
3. *Rotary kilns:* A rotary kiln comprises of a rotating oven and a postcombustion chamber. They are indicated for incineration

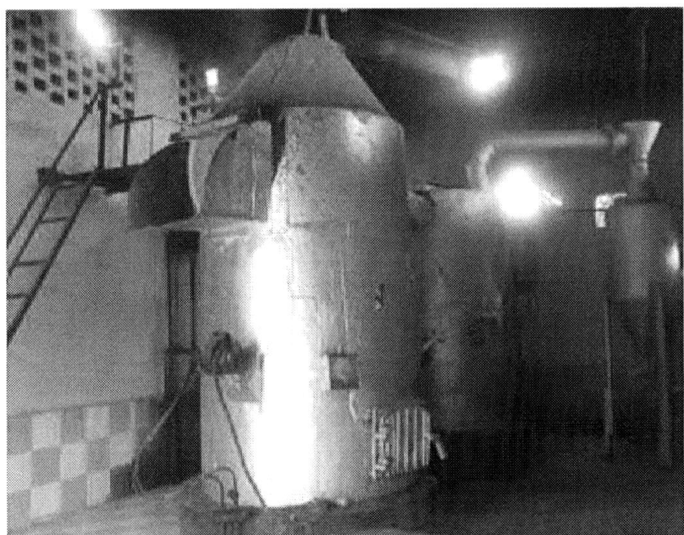

Fig. 10.4: Double chamber pyrolytic chamber
(*Courtesy*: Amritsar Enviro Care System (P) Ltd.)

of chemical wastes (chemicals, pharmaceuticals including cytotoxic drugs).[83]

Monitoring: Monitoring of incinerator should be carried out once in a month to check its performance and to ensure:

- Proper operation and maintenance of the incinerator
- Attainment of prescribed temperatures in primary and secondary chambers of the incinerator during incineration
- No PVC plastics are incinerated
- Only skilled workers operate the incinerator
- Proper record book is maintained for the incinerator which keeps entries of duration of operation, temperature attained during incineration, quantity of waste incinerated, etc.[57]

Disadvantages

1. Incineration proves to be costly because it is very energy intensive process.
2. Biomedical waste incinerators emit dioxins, furans (POPs) (Table 10.5) and heavy metals like mercury, lead and cadmium, fine dust particles, carbon monoxide, hydrogen chloride, sulphur dioxide, nitrogen oxides, Products of Incomplete Combustions (PICs) and many other pollutants into the atmosphere. These hazardous compounds pose serious threat to the health of incineration plant personnel, the public and the environment.
3. Additional equipment or devices to reduce gaseous emissions usually results in increased content of these pollutants in the solid waste phase. Moreover, the filters have a limited efficiency in capturing very fine particles, capturing only 5 to 30 percent of very fine particles smaller than 2.5 µm. The particles less than 1 µm are not captured at all. Recent researches reveal that inhaling these ultrafine particles may adversely affect human health.
4. Incineration ash is also potentially hazardous. The dioxins content in settlings, ash, filter cakes and slag is reported to be 2 percent, 6 percent, 18 percent and 72 percent of the total quantity of released dioxins respectively, as compared to 2 percent in gaseous emissions. The ash also contains high content of heavy metals such as copper, lead, chrome, nickel, zinc.[27]

Table 10.5: The list of Persistent Organic Pollutants (POPs)—the "Dirty Dozen" of 12 toxic chemicals[54]

POP	*Source*
Aldrin and dieldrin	Insecticides used on crops (e.g. corn and cotton) and antitermite solutions.
Chlordane	Insecticide used on crops (e.g. vegetables, small grains, potatoes, sugarcane, sugar beets, fruits, nuts, citrus, and cotton). Also used for termite control. Pesticides used on home lawn and garden pests.
DDT	Insecticide used on agricultural crops (primarily cotton) and insects carrying diseases like malaria and typhus.
Endrin	Insecticide used on crops like cotton and grains. Also used for controlling rodents.
Mirex	Insecticide used to combat termites, fire ants, and mealybugs. Also used for fire retardation in plastics, rubber, and electrical products.
Heptachlor	Insecticide used primarily against soil insects and termites. Also used as a pesticide on some crops and to combat malaria.
Hexachlorobenzene	Fungicide used for treatment of seeds. Also an impurity in certain pesticides. To make fireworks, ammunition, synthetic rubber, and other substances. Also produced during combustion and the manufacture of certain chemicals unintentionally.
PCBs	Used for a variety of industrial processes and purposes, e.g. in electrical transformers and capacitors, as heat exchange fluids, in carbonless copy paper, as paint additives, and in plastics. Also produced as a combustion product unintentionally.
Toxaphene	Insecticide, pesticide for controlling pests on crops and livestock, and to kill unwanted fish in lakes.
Dioxins and furans	Unintentionally produced during combustion of municipal and medical wastes, backyard burning of trash, and industrial processes.
As trace contaminants	In certain herbicides, wood preservatives, and in PCB mixtures.

Source: *Persistent Organic Pollutants: A Global Issue, A Global Response (USEPA).*

Dioxins

Dioxins are easily formed at temperatures between 250 to 450°C.[28] Dioxin formation is believed to be catalyzed by fly ash created during combustion in the presence of metals and a chlorine source. Dioxins are fat-soluble. These can enter the body through fatty foods such as meat and dairy products, e.g. chicken, egg, meat, milk, etc.

It is proven that dioxins can be toxic in very low concentrations. A concentration of 0.006 picogram/kg body weight per day is sufficient to cause toxic effects.[24] According to the International Agency for Research on Cancer (IARC), the most toxic dioxin—2,3,7,8 TCDD is a group 1 human carcinogen. Some other dioxins are also considered possible carcinogenic substances for human beings. Dioxins are also responsible for certain harmful effects on the hormonal system, organism stamina, diabetes, endometriosis and a wide range of other diseases, including genetic defects.

Acid gases: These can have serious respiratory and cardiovascular impacts.

Heavy metals: These can have negative neurological and metabolic impacts.

Controversies about incineration of biomedical waste: The controversies surrounding this process are many.

- The aim of treatment of medical waste is killing pathogens and not destruction of the materials on which the pathogens reside and grow. Incineration destroys both the things
- Incineration of plastics and cellulose rich materials yields a number of harmful products which pollute the environment
- As 85 percent hospital waste is nonhazardous, incineration is not a viable option. So the key to successful management of hospital waste is segregation, not incineration.[23]

Due to rising concerns about deleterious environmental effects of incineration all over the world, a number of newer non-incineration techniques have come up over the time.

Plasma Pyrolysis

Plasma is the state of matter formed by releasing the bound electrons from atoms. It is an electrically conducting fluid which consists of charged and neutral particles. The charged particles possess high kinetic energies. When electrons recombine with ionized species in the plasma, highly energetic ultraviolet radiation is released. This energy changes to heat energy. The charged and excited species make the plasma environment highly reactive, which catalyzes homogeneous and heterogeneous chemical reactions. The end products of plasma pyrolysis of carbonaceous matter are methane, CO, H_2, CO_2 and water molecules.

Plasma pyrolysis utilizes extremely high temperatures of plasma-arc in an oxygen deprived environment to completely decompose waste material into simple molecules. Owing to this property, plasma pyrolysis can be used for treatment of solid waste and destruction of toxic molecules.

Parts of the System

The system consists of the following subsystems:

1. Power supply.
2. Plasma torch.
3. Gas-injection system.
4. Primary reaction chamber.
5. Secondary reaction chamber.
6. Quenching system-cum-scrubber.
7. Induced draft fan.
8. Chimney.

Power Supply

The parameters are:

Power supply—50 KW, DC
Open circuit voltage—400 V
Arc voltage—125 V
Maximum arc current—400 amperes

A high voltage of 3.5 KV and high frequency of 4 MHz are essential to initiate plasma formation in the arc.

Plasma Torch

The plasma torch is made up of a combination of an anode, a cathode and magnetic field. A water cooled tungsten tip surrounded by a copper cup acts as anode. This anode is placed in front of a cathode, and a magnetic field is applied parallel to the axes of anode and cathode. Due to the establishment of arc, both anode and cathode get heated to a temperature of 6727°C and 19727°C respectively.

Gas-injection System

Nitrogen gas is injected through the torch which maintains an oxygen deprived conditions in the chamber and flow of gas is controlled using rotameters.

Process Chamber/Primary Reaction Chamber

The process chamber is tilted and made up of mild steel, and has a waste-feeder, mild-steel shell and glass-wool shielding. The feeder has two doors. The inner one is tightly sealed to prevent leakage of the gas. The outer door prevents spread of gases in the working environment while waste loading is done through inner door.

Secondary Reaction Chamber

In the secondary reaction chamber the gases coming out from the primary reaction chamber pass through a temperature zone of 1050 ± 50°C. These gases are burnt in presence of excess quantity of air and are converted into CO_2 and H_2O. The secondary reaction chamber is designed in such a way that the residence time of the gases is sufficient for complete combustion of gases.

Quenching-cum-scrubbing System

The role of this system of mild steel with ceramic inner lining is to quench the hot gases to inhibit their recombination reactions. NaOH at a pH of 12 and normal temperature is circulated through the chamber with the help of a fountain. NaOH will also remove HCl from the residual gases.

Induced Draft Fan and Chimney

Induced draft fan takes the residual gases at the chimney's height for their release in the atmosphere. It also creates negative pressure in the process chamber and sucks excess air into the secondary chamber.

Advantages

- Even chlorinated wastes and other hazardous wastes need not be segregated
- There is more than 99 percent reduction in volume of organic matter
- The waste is burnt completely without producing any harmful residuals
- The quantity of toxic residuals (dioxins and furans) is much below the accepted emission standards
- The pathogens are completely killed
- There is a possibility to recover energy.[59]

Nonincineration Technologies

Nonincineration treatment technologies can be classified on the basis of fundamental processes used to decontaminate waste. The basic processes are:

1. Thermal processes
2. Chemical processes
3. Irradiative processes
4. Biological processes.

Mechanical processes are used to supplement each of the four fundamental processes.

Thermal Processes

Thermal processes utilize thermal energy or heat to destroy pathogens in the waste. Depending upon the temperature used, thermal processes can be further categorized into low-heat, medium-heat, and high-heat thermal processes.

Low-heat thermal pocesses: Equipments utilizing low-heat thermal processes operate at temperature range of 93 to 177°C (200 to 350°F), which is insufficient to cause chemical breakdown, combustion or pyrolysis.

The two basic categories of low-heat thermal processes are:

- *Dry heat or hot air treatment*: Three basic principles of heat transmission, i.e. conduction, convection (forced or natural) and/or thermal radiation are employed. The waste is disinfected without any steam.

- *Wet heat treatment*: Saturated steam is the mainstay of this treatment. The apparatus used for this purpose can be an autoclave or a microwave.

Medium-heat thermal processes: The two medium heat thermal processes are reverse polymerization (utilizing high-intensity microwave energy) and thermal depolymerization (using heat and high pressure) which take place at temperature range of 177 to 370°C (350 to 700°F). At this temperature, chemical breakdown of organic material occurs without any change in physical appearance of the waste.

High-heat thermal processes: High-heat thermal processes operating at 540 to 8300°C (1,000 to 15,000°F) or higher temperatures bring about chemical and physical changes in both organic and inorganic material resulting in total destruction of the waste as well as 90 to 95 percent reduction in the mass and volume of the waste. Electrical resistance, induction, natural gas, and/or plasma energy are used for this purpose.[27]

Thermal methods are relatively easier to validate and monitor and are less damaging to the environment as compared to chemical treatment.[78]

Chemical Processes

Dissolved chlorine dioxide, NaOCl (bleach), peracetic acid, dry inorganic chemicals, encapsulating compounds, ozone and alkali are various chemical compounds used to disinfect waste.

Irradiative Processes

Irradiation-based technologies utilize electron beams, UV irradiation or cobalt-60 for disinfection of waste. Because irradiation does not alter the waste physically, a grinder or shredder is required to render the waste unrecognizable. Also shielding is mandatory to prevent occupational exposures.

Biological Processes

Enzymes are used to destroy organic matter in such processes.

Mechanical Processes

As above said processes do not render the waste unidentifiable, and also these technologies cannot be fully effective in destroying the microbes due to large size of the waste items. So mechanical processes such as shredding, grinding, hammermill processing, liquid-solid separation, mixing, agitation, conveying, and compaction, etc. are used to supplement these processes.

Advantages of mechanical processes are:

- To increase the contact between waste and disinfectant by increasing the surface area
- To make the body parts unrecognizable and reduce public sensitivity
- To reduce the volume of the waste requiring treatment.

Shredders: Shredders employ high rotational force by means of hardened steel cutting knives, hooks, disks, or blades mounted on slowly rotating shafts. These can be either single-shaft shredders or multiple-shaft shredders (Fig. 10.5).

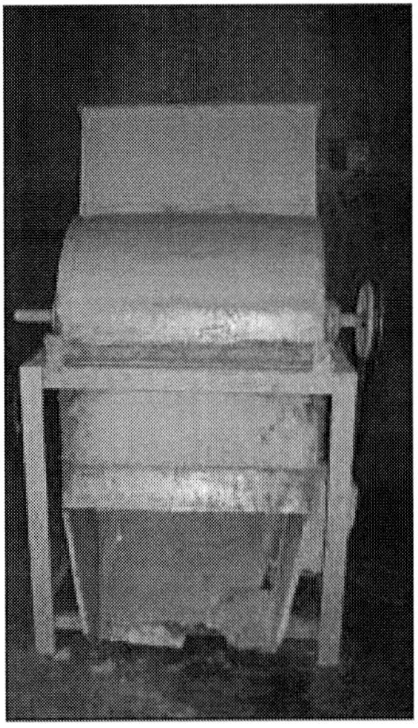
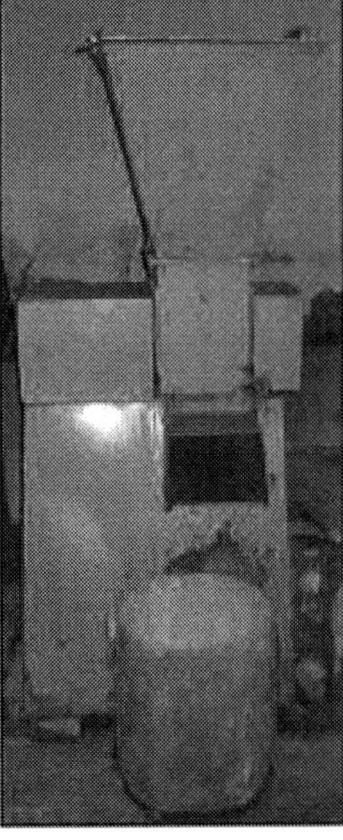

Fig. 10.5: Different types of shredders
(*Courtesy*: Amritsar Enviro Care System (P) Ltd.)

Grinders/crushers/pulverizer: They utilize a series of rollers operating at high speed. The rollers can be equipped with teeth or knives.

Hammermill: In this equipment, steel hammers are attached to a rotating shaft. The shaft rotating at high speed crushes waste with the hammers against a plate.

All these devices require intensive maintenance. Hammers need to be periodically resurfaced, cutting knives need to be sharpened, and worn or broken shredder blades need to be replaced.

Detailed description of the above-mentioned waste treatment processes is as follows:

Low-heat Thermal Technologies

Autoclave

An autoclave is a metallic device with metal chamber, outer steam jacket and sealed by a charging door (Fig. 10.6). Steam is introduced into both the outside jacket and the inside chamber which can withstand very high pressures. The role of heated outside jacket is to reduce condensation in the inside chamber wall and allow the

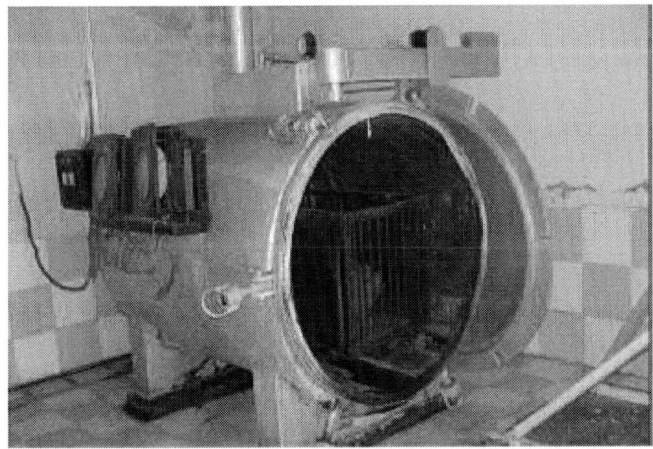

Fig. 10.6: Waste autoclave
(*Courtesy*: Amritsar Enviro Care System (P) Ltd.)

use of steam at lower temperatures. Air being an insulator can hamper with the penetration of heat into the waste. Based on the method of removal of air, autoclaves are of two types:

a. Gravity displacement or downward-displacement autoclave
b. Prevacuuming or high-vacuum autoclave.

Steam, being lighter than air, forces the air downward into an outlet port or drain line in the lower part of the chamber in a gravity-displacement autoclave. Whereas in a prevacuum autoclave, a vacuum pump is used to evacuate air before introducing steam. It is better than gravity-displacement autoclave as prevacuum autoclaves need less time for disinfection.

Treatment cycle of an autoclave:

i. *Waste collection*: Waste is collected in containers lined with autoclavable liner.
ii. *Preheating of autoclave*: Steam is introduced into the outer jacket of the autoclave.
iii. *Waste loading*: Waste containers are loaded into the inside chamber. To monitor disinfection, chemical or biological indicators are periodically placed in the middle of the waste load. The charging door is then closed to seal the chamber.[28] When solid containers (e.g. buckets) have been placed in the autoclave they should be uncovered. Their depth should not exceed 9 inches, and autoclave bags should be opened so that air is removed and steam penetration occurs. Because if bags are left closed, the retained air will depress the temperature and contents will be subjected to dry heat and at such low temperatures, dry heating is not an effective method for sterilization.
iv. *Air evacuation*: Complete evacuation of air is must for attaining correct temperature within the autoclave.[27] It ensures that a uniform internal pressure of 15 lb/in^2 or (1.01×10^5 N/m^2) and temperature of 121°C is attained. Containers used for autoclaving laboratory waste must not hinder the process of air evacuation from the chamber as it may lower the temperature. Air is evacuated through either gravity displacement or prevacuuming.[76]

v. *Steam treatment*: Introduction and continued induction of steam into the chamber serves two purposes—First, it raises the chamber temperature to required reading. Second, it helps to maintain this temperature for required duration.[27] Recommended parameters for autoclaving are:

I. In a gravity flow autoclave, medical waste should be subjected to:

i. Temperature—not less than 121°C
Pressure—15 psi
Autoclave residence time—not less than 60 minutes; or

ii. Temperature—not less than 135°C
Pressure—31 psi
Autoclave residence time—not less than 45 minutes; or

iii. Temperature—not less than 149°C
Pressure of 52 psi
Autoclave residence time—not less than 30 minutes

II. In a vacuum autoclave, medical waste should be subjected to a minimum of one prevacuum pulse to evacuate all the air from the autoclave. Then the waste should be subjected to:

i. Temperature—not less than 121°C
Pressure—5 psi
Autoclave residence time -not less than 45 minutes; or

ii. Temperature—not less than 135°C
Pressure—31 psi
Autoclave residence time—not less than 30 minutes.

Medical waste should be considered properly treated only when the time, temperature and pressure indicators indicate that the required time, temperature and pressure were reached during the autoclave process. If for any reasons this is not ensured, the entire load of medical waste must be autoclaved again until the standard parameters of temperature, pressure and residence time are achieved.[52] In addition to these parameters, microbial inactivation must be tested through appropriate validation tests[27] (see *Microbial Inactivation*).

vi. *Steam discharge:* Steam is released to reduce the pressure and temperature, in the chamber, usually through a condenser.

vii. *Unloading:* The waste is allowed to cool down further and the treated waste is removed. The indicator strips are removed and evaluated.

viii. *Mechanical treatment:* To render the waste unrecognizable and suitable for disposal in a landfill, a shredder or compactor is used.[27]

Load Types

Autoclaves are used to treat:

Autoclaves are used to sterilize several different types of loads:

Solid—Metal, glass, plastic, sharps

Porous—Linen, gowns, paper, gauze, bandages, drapes, beddings, complex instruments, hollow tubes, materials contaminated with blood and limited amounts of fluids, isolation and surgery wastes.

Liquid—Water, saline, media, cultures and stocks.

Laboratory waste—Petridishes, sample bottles, syringes (excluding chemical waste).[85]

Waste Types not to be Treated

- Volatile and semivolatile organic compounds
- Mercury and other heavy metals
- Chemotherapeutic wastes
- Other hazardous chemical wastes
- Radiological wastes.

Waste loads that block the transfer of heat such as large animal carcasses huge and bulky bedding material, sealed heat-resistant containers, should also be avoided.

Emissions and Waste Residues

i. *Odor*: Foul odor is a problem around autoclaves and retorts if sufficient ventilation is not provided in the treatment area. If there is insufficient ventilation, odors can be a problem around autoclaves and retorts.

ii. *Toxic contaminants:* If antineoplastic drugs or heavy metals, etc. are autoclaved along with other wastes, toxic contaminants will be released into the air, condensate or in the treated waste itself.

iii. Emission of low levels of alcohol, phenols, aldehydes, and other organic compounds in the air has been recorded, e.g. 2-propanol measured at 643 mg/m^3 in vicinity of the operating autoclave.

Microbial Inactivation

A number of chemical indicators or biological monitors are available which are placed at the center of test loads. If sufficient to verify that sufficient steam penetration and exposure have occurred, either color of the indicator will change or the microbes will be inactivated at the end of treatment cycle.[27]

Validation Tests

Spore Test

The autoclave should completely and consistently kill the approved biological indicator at the maximum design capacity of each autoclave unit. Biological indicator for autoclave shall be *Bacillus stearothermophilus* spores using vials or spore strips; with at least 1 × 10000 spores per ml. An autoclave should never be operated below the minimum operating parameters, i.e.

- Residence time of 30 minutes, regardless of temperature and pressure
- Temperature of 121°C or
- Pressure of 15 psi.

Routine Test

A chemical indicator strip/tape that changes color when a certain temperature is reached can be used to verify the required specific temperature. It is recommended to use more than one strip over the waste package and at a different location to ensure that the inner content of the package has been adequately autoclaved.[52]

Advantages of the Autoclave

Autoclaves and retorts have the following advantages:

- Saturated steam treatment is a proven sterilization technology. Hence, a popular method for BMW treatment all over the world
- The technology is easy to understand, easy to operate and hence readily accepted by hospital staff and communities
- Time-temperature parameters for sterilization are well-established
- Available in wide range of capacity as per requirement
- The emissions from autoclaves and retorts are minimal, in well-segregated wastes
- Relatively low capital costs.

Disadvantages

The disadvantages include:

- The treated waste is still recognizable in the absence of a shredder or grinder
- Offensive odors can be generated if proper air ventilation is not taken care of
- In case hazardous chemicals (e.g. mercury, cytotoxic agents, formaldehyde or phenol) are present in the waste, these toxic contaminants can be released into the air, wastewater, or remain in the residue to contaminate the landfill
- In the absence of a method of drying the waste, condensed steam makes the treated waste is heavier than the untreated input waste
- Direct contact with steam is mandatory. So if barriers to direct steam exposure or heat transfer are present, disinfection will be incomplete.

Microwave System

Microwave disinfection is a steam-based process in which disinfection occurs through the action of moist heat and steam generated by microwave energy.

Microwaves are waves with very short wavelengths, falling between Ultrahigh Frequency (UHF) used for television and the infrared range in the electromagnetic spectrum. Microwave systems consist of a microwave generator (magnetron) which directs the microwave energy into a disinfection area or chamber. In general, 2 to 6 magnetrons are used with an output of about 1.2 kW each. These systems may be designed as batch processes or semicontinuous.

How it Works

High-temperature steam is injected into the hopper; air is extracted through a HEPA filter. Then waste is loaded into the hopper and its flap is closed. Upon closing the flap, internal shredding of waste begins to break it into smaller particles. 4 to 6 MW generators heat the shredded waste to 95 to 100°C for a minimum of total 30 minutes. Then this treated waste is discharged into a bin/container by means of a conveyer screw. Thereafter the bins may be sent for compaction or sanitary landfill.

Types of Waste Treated

The similar types of waste treated in autoclaves and retorts can be treated in microwave systems. Indications and contraindications for waste types also remain the same.

Emissions and Waste Residues

The problem of odor in microwave technology is almost the same as in autoclave. No volatile organic compounds were found in vicinity of microwave treatment units whereas level of 2-propanol near the autoclave facility was measured at 2318 mg/m^3.

Microbial Inactivation

Microwave treatment can destroy the following test organisms:

Staphylococcus aureus, Candida albicans, Mycobacterium bovis, Bacillus subtilis, Enterococcus faecalis, Pseudomonas aeruginosa, Mycobacterium fortuitum, Nocardia asteroides, Aspergillus fumigatus, Giardia miura and duck hepatitis.

Advantages of the Technology

Advantages of microwave technology include the following:

- Hospital staff and communities can easily to understand and accept the technology
- Proper segregation can minimize the toxic emissions well below the detection limit
- The technology is automated, easy to use and require only one operator.

Disadvantages

The disadvantages are:

- In poorly segregated wastes, hazardous chemicals in the waste can be released into the air or remain in the waste to contaminate the landfill.
- Some offensive odors around the microwave unit may be present.
- The secondary shredder used for sharps is a bit noisy.
- The shredder could get damaged due to any large, hard metal object in the waste.
- Relatively high capital cost.[27]

Hydroclave

The Hydroclave Process and How It Works

The hydroclave is essentially a double-walled (jacketed) cylindrical, pressurized vessel, horizontally mounted, with one or more side or top loading doors, and a smaller unloading door at the bottom. The very small hydroclave units have a single side door for both loading and unloading.

The vessel is fitted with a motor driven shaft, to which are attached powerful fragmenting/mixing arms that slowly rotate inside the vessel.

When steam is introduced in the vessel jacket, it transmits heat rapidly to the fragmented waste, which, in turn, produces steam of its own.

A temperature sensor is located in the bottom inside part of the vessel, which measures the temperature of the waste as it is agitated and mixed, and this sensor reports back to the main computerized controller, which automatically sets treatment parameters ensuring complete waste sterility—even liquid infectious waste.

After sterilization, the liquid but sterile components of the waste, are steamed out of the vessel, recondensed and drained to sewer. The remaining waste is dehydrated, fragmented, and self-unloaded via a reverse rotation of the mixer/agitator.

In summary, the hydroclave:

- Sterilizes the waste utilizing steam, similar to an autoclave, but with much faster and much more even heat penetration.
- Hydrolyzes the organic components of the waste such as pathological material.
- Removes the water content (dehydrates) the waste.
- Breaks up the waste into small pieces of fragmented material.
- Reduces the waste substantially in weight and volume.
- Accomplishes the above within the totally sealed vessel, which is not opened until all waste it totally sterile.

There is no correlation between waste characteristics and treatment efficacy. All the waste is consistently sterilized.

Liquid and heavy loads, however, will take somewhat longer to reach the temperature and pressure required to initiate the sterilization cycle, but sterilization automatically occurs.

There is no need for "pre- and postvacuum", that is, pull infectious air and liquids of the vessel, as is the case with autoclaves. Pulling air and liquids out of an infectious environment increases the risk of live pathogen emission.

The hydroclave eliminates this risk due to the vigorous dynamic activity within the hydroclave, which mixes and heats any entrained air with the steam and waste material.

Detailed Description of the Treatment Cycle

Loading (Fig. 10.7)

The waste can be loaded into the hydroclave treatment vessel by various means, depending on your requirements:

- In smaller units dropping the waste bags manually into a side or end door
- In medium-sized units by tipping waste containers into top or angled loading doors. Electric or hydraulic tipping devices are an available option with the hydroclave
- In medium to large sized units, for large scale commercial operation, a combination of conveyors, hoppers and tippers are available to load the waste into large top loading doors.

The hydroclave can be fitted with loading doors to suit your requirements, from small side doors to multiple angled or top

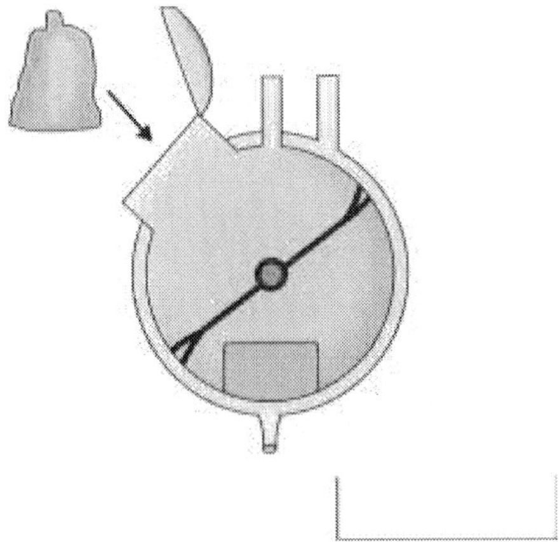

Fig. 10.7: Loading in hydroclave

doors, which are sized to accommodate your infectious waste stream-small doors for bagged biomedical waste, to very large doors for disinfecting large objects such as large animal carcasses.

No special operator skill is required, since overloading or loading too tightly is not an issue with this type of process.

Heat-up and Fragmentation (Fig. 10.8)

After loading, the vessel doors are closed, and the outer jacket of the vessel is filled with high-temperature steam, which acts as an indirect heating medium for heating the waste.

The jacket steam condenses into clean, hot condensate, which is returned back to the steam boiler. This unique feature makes the hydroclave so efficient in operation—no steam or hot condensate is lost.

During heat-up, the shaft and mixing arms rotate, causing the waste to be fragmented and continuously tumbled against the hot vessel walls.

At this point, the waste is broken up into small fragments, and all material heats-up rapidly, being evenly and thoroughly exposed to the hot inner surfaces. The moisture content of the waste will turn to steam, and the vessel will start to pressurize.

Initially, no steam will be injected into the waste. If there is not enough moisture in the waste to pressurize the vessel, a small

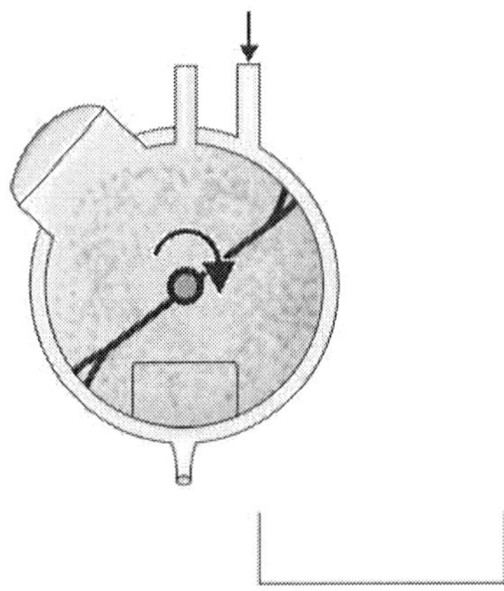

Fig. 10.8: Heat-up and fragmentation

amount of boiler steam is added until the desired pressure is reached.

The uniform jacket heat, and the location of the temperature sensor ensures that even liquid waste will be heated up uniformly.

At the end of this period, the correct sterilization temperature and pressure are reached, and the sterilization period is initiated automatically.

Sterilization Period (Fig. 10.9)

By computer or PLC control, the temperature and pressure are maintained for the desired time to achieve sterilization. If for any reason the sterilization parameters drop below desired levels, the sterilization cycle is stopped, and reinitiated. This ensures sterilization prior to commencement of the next stage.

The mixing/fragmenting arms continue to rotate during the entire sterilization period, to ensure thorough heat penetration into each waste particle.

As independently tested by the University of Ottawa, Dept. of Microbiology, a sterilization time of 15 minutes at 132°C, or 30 minutes at 121°C. achieves 6log10 inactivation of the spores of *Bacillus stearothermophilus*.

The intense subjugation of the waste to such temperature and pressure moisture in a dynamic environment will also cause the

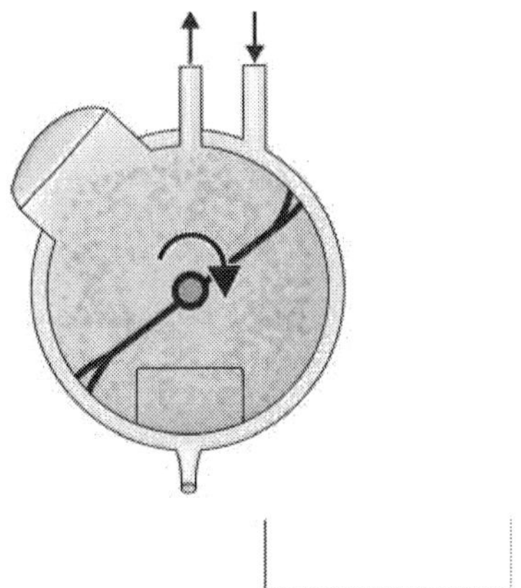

Fig. 10.9: Sterilization period

waste to hydrolyze, that is a rapid decomposition of organic waste material.

Depressurization and Dehydration

After the sterilization period ends, the vessel is depressurized via a steam condenser, which causes initial waste dehydration due to depressurization.

The steam to the jacket will remain on, agitation continues, and the waste loses its remaining water content through a combination of heat input from the jacket and continued agitation.

All waste, no matter how wet initially, even liquid waste, will be dehydrated by this process.

Unloading (Fig. 10.10)

At the end of the depressurization/dehydration period, jacket steam is shut off, the discharge door is opened, and the powerful mixing arms are reversed to a clockwise rotation.

Due to the unique construction of the mixing arms, the opposite rotation causes the fragmented waste to be pushed out of the vessel discharge door, into a waste container, or onto a conveyor.

If desired, the waste can be further fine-shredded prior to final disposal, by a separate shredding system. The dry, sterile, fragmented waste is well suited for further fine shredding.

The vessel is now ready for another treatment cycle, having retained most of its heat for the treatment of the next batch.[42]

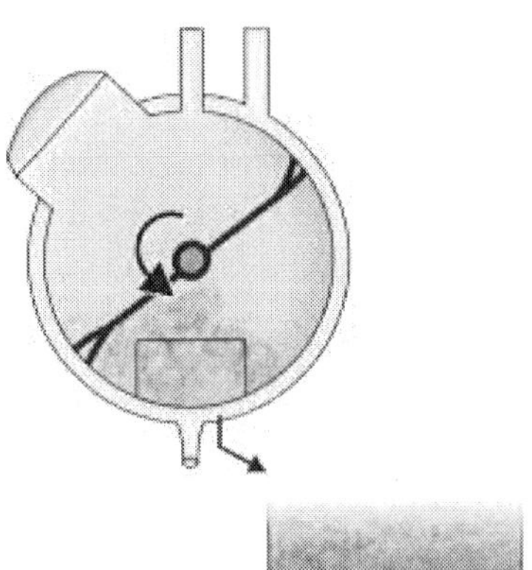

Fig. 10.10: Unloading

Advantages

- Hydroclave provides guaranteed sterilization of the waste to 6 Log 10 spore reduction, ensuring total kill of organisms, even heat-resistant *Bacillus stearothermophilus*, HIV and HBV
- As the liquid effluent is sterile, it can be safely disposed through the sanitary sewer
- It has no harmful emissions into the environment and is well within the Occupational Exposure Limits of the WHO
- As it retains heat for next load, it has the lowest operating cost among autoclaves
- Vacuum pumps, HEPA filters, expensive plastic bags and special carts or bins are not required
- Recycling of hot condensate from the jacket to the boiler feed tank makes it 30 percent cheaper to operate by saving water
- PVCs and chlorinated products can be treated in a hydroclave as it operates at low temperatures and pressures. It does not even produce any dioxins or furans
- The residual waste is safe for recycling or landfilling.[43]

Few instructions about efficient use of steam treatment units:

1. For each steam treatment unit, a current written operating procedure must be available which should specify, at a minimum, the following:
   a. Parameters that provide consistent treatment such as exposure time, temperature, and pressure.
   b. Standardized containers for waste loading and their placement in the steam treatment unit.
2. The steam treatment units must be regularly serviced to prevent any sort of functional irregularities. The service record should always be available on-site.
3. After treatment of biomedical waste, only a permitted and certified waste transport service company should be allowed to pick up the waste for disposal.
4. It is recommended to maintain a written log for each steam treatment unit. Every time the unit is used, the following should be recorded:
   a. The date, time of operation and operator's name.
   b. The type and tentative wt. or vol. of waste treated.

c. The post-treatment confirmation results by either:
   i. Recording the temperature, pressure, and duration of waste treatment or
   ii. Temperature and pressure indicator devices.
d. Dates and results of calibration and maintenance.
e. The results of sterilization indicators, such as *B. stearothermophilus* or equivalent.[25]

Chemical Processes

- The chlorine-based chemical disinfectants were the most commonly used chemical methods for treating medical waste in the past, because of the ability of chlorine and hypochlorite to kill a broad range of microorganisms. However, nonchlorine chemical disinfectants are now available, e.g. peroxyacetic acid (peracetic acid).
- Glutaraldehyde
- Ozone gas
- Sodium hydroxide
- Calcium oxide.

Types of Waste Treated

The following types of waste are commonly treated in chemical-based technologies:

Cultures and stocks, liquid human and animal wastes including blood and body fluids, sharps, isolation and surgery wastes, soft wastes such as gauze, bandages, drapes, gowns, bedding, etc. from patient care and laboratory waste (except chemical waste).

Wastes Which will not to be Treated

Volatile and semivolatile organic compounds, mercury, chemotherapeutic wastes, other hazardous chemical wastes, and radiological wastes.

Emissions and Waste Residues

During shredding, pathogens may release into environment through aerosol formation. Occupational exposures to the chemical disinfectants through fugitive emissions, accidental leaks or spills from storage containers, discharges from the treatment unit, chemical vapors from treated waste or liquid effluent, etc. are also a cause of concern.

Microbial Inactivation

Vegetative bacteria and fungi, fungal spores, and lipophilic viruses are easily destroyed by chemical-based technologies. However hydrophilic viruses, mycobacteria, and bacterial spores such as *B. stearothermophilus* are more resistant to these methods.

Advantages of the Technology

- Well-understood, accepted and approved process since many years (particularly sodium hypochlorite)
- Well-automated and easy to use technology
- Liquid effluents can be discharged into the sanitary sewer
- No combustion by products
- The waste is rendered unrecognizable by shredding.

Disadvantages

The disadvantages are:

- Possible toxic by products in the waste water from large scale chlorine and hypochlorite systems
- Chemical hazards
- Hazardous chemicals, if present in the waste, are released into the air and wastewater or remain in the waste to contaminate the landfill. They may also react with the chemical disinfectant to form other compounds that may or may not be hazardous
- Some offensive odors around some chemical treatment units are noticed.[27]

Details about the Chemicals Used

Ozone

Ozone is a triatomic molecule of oxygen (O_3). As ozone is an unstable, molecule it changes to O_2 within approx. half an hour under normal atmospheric conditions.

Due to this property of releasing nascent oxygen, ozone is a powerful oxidizing agent. It can oxidize a number of molecules including metals (except gold, platinum, and iridium), nitrogen oxides, carbon, ammonia, and sulfides. It can oxidize C=C bonds which is the basic bond in various biological molecules and most of pharmaceuticals. Resultantly, ozone can destroy essentially all pathogens, i.e. bacteria, fungi, viruses, as well as prions.

Ozone can be easily generated on site using simple technology, and thus unlike other chemicals, does not require specialized containers for transport. Further, ozone does not leave any toxic residue behind as it degrades naturally into oxygen.

Use of Ozone as a Disinfectant

Ozone can be used for water treatment for drinking purposes, disinfecting medical instruments as well as for the treatment of biomedical waste. However it can be used only as a method for topical sterilization because it cannot shred the materials.

However, ozonator system combines waste treatment with shredding, thus increasing the effectiveness of the process. It works on the basis of a continuous batch process, and each batch of a maximum 200 kg load requires about 10 minutes for processing. The system operates at a power supply of 37 kW (peak). The entire process is fully automated (loading, shredding, ozone treatment and unloading), hence reduces the exposure of workers. The treatment phase works at ozone levels of 3500 to 4500 ppm.

Microbial Inactivation

One hour treatment with ozone results in reduction in viability of Bacillus atrophaeus and *Geobacillus stearothermophilus* spores. *Bacillus subtilis* ATCC 9372 spores also show reduction in spore viability under standard conditions of treatment. It is reported to be effective in killing 99.9999 percent of microorganisms. After processing, waste is suitable for removal to a landfill site.[71]

Sodium Hypochlorite (NaOCl) (Tables 10.6 and 10.7)

A 3 to 6 percent concentration of sodium hypochlorite effectively destroys in bacteria, fungi, and viruses, and in controlling odor.

Table 10.6: Dilution of sodium hypochlorite and available chlorine

Sodium hypochlorite concentration	*Dilution*	*Chlorine (ppm)*
5.25 to 6.15%	No dilution	52,500 to 61,500
	1:10	5,250 to 6,150
	1:100	525 to 615
	1:1000	53 to 62

Source: *Guideline for Disinfection and Sterilization in Healthcare Facility, 2008.*

Table 10.7: Chlorine releasing compounds used for disinfection of items contaminated with blood and body fluids

Chlorine releasing disinfectant	*Available chlorine*	*Required chlorine*	*Contact period*	*Disinfectant per 1 L water*
Sodium hypochlorite	5%	0.5%	30 minutes	100 ml
Calcium hypochlorite	70%	0.5%	30 minutes	7 g
Sodium dichlorosoc-yanurate (powder)	----	0.5%	30 minutes	8.5 g
Sodium hypochlorite tablets	----	0.5%	30 minutes	4 tablets
Chloramine	25%	0.5%	30 minutes	20 g

Source: *Singh Z, Bhalwar R, Jayaram J, Tilak VW. An Introduction to Bio-medical Waste Management.*

Disadvantages

- Reactions between chlorine or hypochlorite and organic matter produce toxic trihalomethanes, haloacetic acids and chlorinated aromatic compounds.
- It can irritate the respiratory tract, skin and eyes.

Chlorine Dioxide

It is an unstable gas that decomposes to form toxic chlorine gas and heat in presence of air. It is stable as a dilute aqueous solution. It has the same biocidal effect as that of chlorine and hypochlorite. It is effective and safe at a concentration of 0.1 ppm. However, proper ventilation and self-contained breathing apparatus is recommended in the operating area.

It does not form toxic compounds by reacting with organic matter. Rather it decomposes to form salts.[27]

Ethylene Oxide

Ethylene oxide (a carcinogen) is used as a fumigant or sterilant in hospitals, medical and dental clinics. It is a gaseous sterilant used for heat-sensitive medical equipment, surgical instruments, and other objects and fluids coming in contact with biological tissues. It can also be used for disinfection of plastics, e.g. catheters to render them reusable.[32]

Ethylene oxide (EtO) gas works at relatively low temperatures for sterilization. If a heated unit is used, sterilization can be achieved in 2 to 3 hours at 120°F. However, after each cycle, a lengthy aeration time is must.[31]

Occupational exposure may occur in following conditions:

1. Leakage from valves, fittings, piping, and sterilizer door gaskets.
2. From opening of the sterilizer door at the end of a cycle.
3. While changing pressurized gas cylinders containing EtO.
4. Due to improper ventilation at the sterilizer door and from inadequate general room ventilation.
5. From improperly or unventilated air gap between the discharge line and the sewer drain.
6. While removing items from the sterilizer and transferring the sterilized load to an aerator.
7. From passing near operating sterilizers and aerators.[32]

Advantages

- Since water content is only 15 percent, no corrosion, rusting, and dulling of instruments occurs
- No destruction of dental items, such as endodontic files, wires and bands, burs, orthodontic pliers, and carbon steel instruments
- Instruments are dry at the end of the cycle.

Disadvantage

- Requirement for adequate ventilation.[21]

According to OSHA

- Permissible Exposure Limit (PEL) = 1 ppm
- Acceptable Peak Exposure = 5 ppm (15-minute excursion).[32]

Irradiation Technologies

Irradiation technologies include electron beam systems, UV irradiation, Cobalt-60, etc. The radiation used in these technologies can be ionizing, (e.g. X-rays and gamma rays) or nonionizing radiation (e.g. microwaves and visible light). Ionizing radiation acts by causing extensive damage to DNA or by producing free radicals that cause further damage by reacting with macromolecules in the cell (e.g. proteins, enzymes, etc.) leading to cell death.[27]

Cobalt-60 is a deliberately produced radioactive isotope. Pencil-like rods of nonradioactive cobalt-59 are bombarded with neutrons in a nuclear reactor for one or more years. This converts about 10 percent of the cobalt-59 into cobalt-60. The pencils are then removed from the reactor and further processed.

The cobalt-60 is used to treat sludge in water treatment units. It emits gamma rays during its decay to nickel. As these gamma rays pass through sludge, they kill microorganisms and parasites. They neither leave any residue in or on the sludge nor make the sludge "radioactive". This irradiation process does not have any effect on moisture content, the levels of nutrients, heavy metals, etc.[87]

UV-C or Ultraviolet Radiation

UV radiation in C range wavelength 2537 Å is also known as germicidal or short wave UV.

UV-C can be effectively used to destroy aerosolized pathogens from shredders and other mechanical devices.

Electron Beam Technology

The e-beam technology does not use any radioactive sources and does not have residual radiation after turning off the e-beam system. However it may induce radioactivity if very high energies are used, e.g. above 10 or 16 MeV). But some concerns have been raised that low levels of radioactivity may be induced at much lower energies.

How it Works

E-beam technologies require minimal handling as these are highly automated and computer controlled. These e-beam systems generally consist of:

- A power supply
- A beam accelerator to generate, accelerate and direct the electrons towards the target
- A scanning system to deliver the required dose
- A cooling system for cooling the accelerator and other assemblies
- A vacuum system to maintain a vacuum in the accelerator;
- A shield for protection of workers
- A conveyor system for transportation of the waste
- Sensors and controls.

E-beams do not alter the waste physically. So shredders or other mechanical device are required in the postprocessing stage to reduce waste volume and render the waste unrecognizable.

Types of Waste Treated

The types of waste commonly treated in an e-beam technology are:

- Cultures and stocks
- Sharps
- Laboratory waste (excluding chemical waste)
- Materials contaminated with blood and body fluids
- Isolation and surgery wastes and
- Soft wastes (bandages, gauzes, gowns, drapes, bedding, etc.) from patient care.

Waste Types not to be Treated

Volatile and semivolatile organic compounds, chemotherapeutic wastes, heavy metals, e.g. mercury, other hazardous chemical wastes, and radiological wastes should not be treated in e-beam units.

Emissions and Waste Residues

E-beam systems do not produce any pollutant emissions except for small amounts of ozone which breaks down to O_2 eventually. This residual ozone removes odors and supplements the disinfection process.

Microbial Inactivation

B. stearothermophilus and *B. subtilis* spores are inactivated by irradiation where as *B. pumilus* spores and *Deinococcus radiodurans* are resistant to irradiation.

Advantages of the Technology

Advantages of e-beam treatment technologies include the following:

- The basic technology is familiar to hospital staff involved in cancer therapy
- No toxic emissions (except for small amounts of ozone) and liquid effluents are produced
- No ionizing radiations are produced after turning the machine off
- It is a low temperature process and requires no steam, water, chemicals, heat, etc
- The technology is well-automated and requires no handling and little operator time
- It has a low operating cost.

Disadvantages of the Technology

The disadvantages include:

- Personnel need protection from radiation exposure
- The e-beam system requires a several feet thick concrete shield or an underground structure, which adds significantly to the installation capital cost
- Ozone off-gas needs to be removed before releasing the exhaust to the atmosphere
- The technology itself does not reduce waste volume or render the waste unrecognizable.[27]

LANDFILL

There are two different types of waste disposal to land—*Open dumping* and *Sanitary landfills.*

Open Dumping

It means uncontrolled and scattered deposition of wastes at a site. This causes higher risks of disease transmission, acute pollution problems, fires and open access to scavengers and animals. Healthcare waste carries the risk of disease transmission through contact, inhalation, or ingestion, or indirectly through the food chain or pathogenic organisms and vectors of diseases. Hence, it should never be disposed in open dumps.

Sanitary Landfills

A small 2 m deep burial pit is prepared to receive healthcare waste only. It should be filled to a depth of 1 to 1.5 m. The bottom of the pit should be at least 1.5 meters above the groundwater level. After dumping each waste load, the waste should be covered with a 10 to 15 cm thick soil or lime layer. There should be restricted access to this dedicated disposal area. The use of a fence around the pit would prevent scavenging by making supervision by landfill staff easier. The safety of waste burial depends critically on rational operational practices.

Atypical example of pit design for healthcare waste is shown in the advantages of sanitary landfills over open dumping are:

- Isolation of wastes from the environment
- Well-planned site to accept wastes
- On-site staff to control operations
- Organized deposit and daily coverage of waste.

Sanitary landfill prevents contamination of soil, surface water and groundwater, and limits air pollution, smells, and direct contact with the public. The following points should always be kept in mind:

- Only hazardous healthcare waste should be buried in a sanitary landfill. Otherwise, general hospital waste would quickly fill up the available space.
- Only small quantities (not more than 1 kg) of chemical wastes should be buried at one time. It avoids serious problems of environmental pollution.
- Each layer of waste should be covered with a layer of soil to prevent odors and proliferation of rodents and insects.[66]

CHAPTER

11 Dental Office Wastes

A number of biomedical wastes including sharps, blood soaked materials and human tissue are produced in dental office. The dental community should ensure that these biomedical wastes are disposed safely to protect human health and the environment.[28] The dentists should be conversant with the disposal of biomedical wastes (Management and Handling) Rules, 1998.[45]

TYPES OF HAZARDOUS DENTAL WASTES

1. Mercury containing wastes
   a. Elemental mercury
   b. Scrap amalgam
2. Silver containing wastes
   a. Spent X-ray fixer
   b. Undeveloped film
3. Lead containing wastes
   a. Lead foil packets
   b. Lead aprons
4. Biomedical wastes
   a. Anatomical biomedical wastes (human tissue)
   b. Nonanatomical biomedical wastes (blood soaked materials)
   c. Sharps
5. Chemicals, disinfectants and sterilizing agents.

MERCURY CONTAINING 7WASTES

Disposal Options

Elemental Mercury

Mercury is toxic to the environment when released. Liquid elemental mercury should be replaced with precapsulated amalgam.

Best Management Practice (BMP)

Always keep unused elemental mercury stored in a tightly sealed, break resistant, labeled container. Label the container as "Hazardous Waste: Elemental Mercury."

Cautions

- Do not throw elemental mercury in the garbage.
- Do not discard elemental mercury down the drain.[10]
- Do not discard elemental mercury in the trash.
- Do not put elemental mercury in the sharps container.
- Do not discard as yellow bag waste.[61]

Use of mercury in the healthcare sector (Equipments and materials):

- Thermometers (Fig. 11.1) (One clinical thermometer contains 0.5 to 1.5 gm of mercury*)
- Sphygmomanometers (Fig. 11.2)
- Feeding tubes
- Dilators and batteries
- Dental amalgam
- Fluorescent tubes

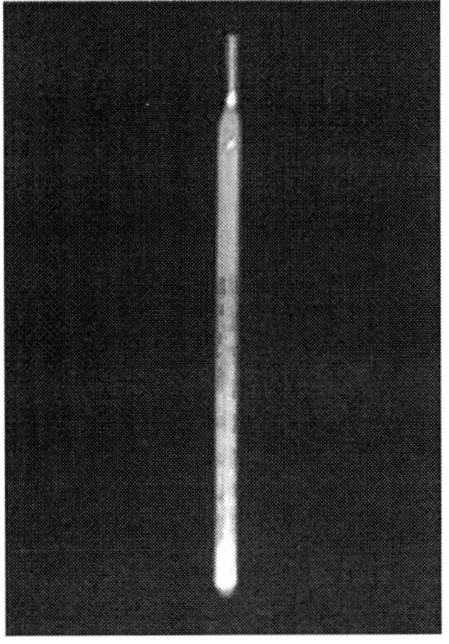

Fig. 11.1: Conventional thermometer

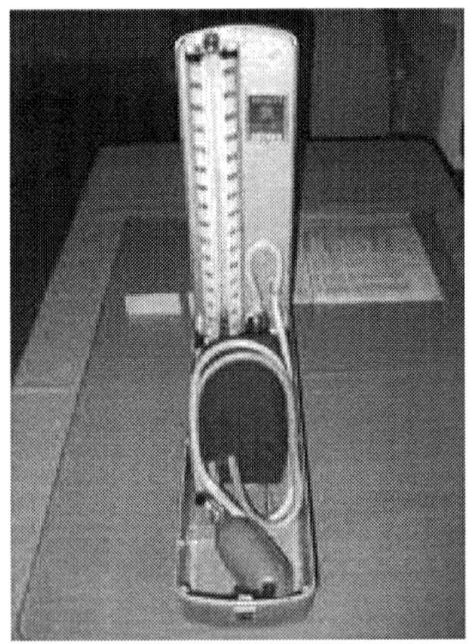

Fig. 11.2: Conventional sphygmomanometer

**One gram of mercury can contaminate a lake of 20 acres*

- Certain laboratory chemicals like Zenker's solution and histological fixatives.

Health hazards of mercury

Mercury can pass through all the three delicately designed barriers in living animals—the skin, blood brain barrier and the placental barrier. Its portal of entry into the body can be:

a. Consumption via food
b. Inhalation or absorption through the skin.[2,58]

Its average half-life in human body is 55 days.[74] Mercury exposure can lead to some clinical conditions namely personality changes, irritability, muscle tremors, gingivitis, bronchitis, pneumonitis, and other forms of nerve damage.

Mercury also affects the central nervous system resulting in:

- Insomnia
- Attention deficit
- Tremors
- Impaired vision and hearing
- Paralysis
- Fetal developmental deficits and delayed development during childhood.

It is particularly dangerous to women of childbearing age, pregnant women, fetuses and young children. Mercury can affect environment in two ways:

1. Hg in water bodies $\xrightarrow{\text{In presence of bacteria}}$ methyl-mercury → fish → food chain
2. A more acidic environment increases organic mercury (a form of mercury) which is easily absorbed by fish, thus making the situation worse.

Mercury is considered a global pollutant as it travels long distances, carried by wind and rain. Mercury does not breakdown; rather it accumulates in the muscles of animals, concentrating as it moves up the food chain.[2,58]

The threat of a mercury spill is highest in dental offices where elemental mercury is used. So, to eliminate the chances of mercury spill, switch to precapsulated amalgam. As a safeguard, all dental offices should be equipped with a mercury spill kit.[10]

Mercury Containment Kit (Fig. 11.3)

a. Face mask
b. Protective eyewear
c. Nitrile gloves or at least two pairs of latex gloves (mercury passes through a single pair of latex gloves)
d. Scotch tape
e. 10 cc syringe
f. Covered plastic container with water
g. Posters depicting the process of mercury spill containment.

Precautions

Avoid using carpets in dental office. If a mercury spill occurs, do as follows:

- Remove all ornaments while dealing with mercury as mercury combines with gold, silver and other metals
- Clear the area around the spill
- Limit the spread of mercury and use two hard cardboard sheets to gather all the droplets of spilled mercury.

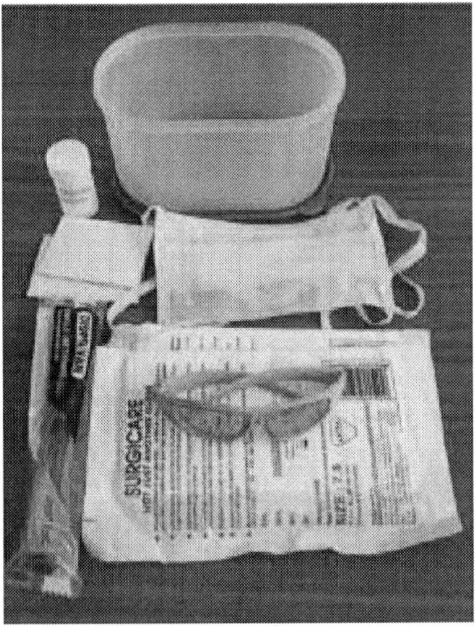

Fig. 11.3: Mercury containment kit

- Suck up mercury with a syringe. Minor mercury spills can be gathered by using stiff paper to scoop it or by using the sticky end of a scotch tape. Since mercury is a nonwetting liquid and has an affinity for its own molecules, small droplets of mercury join to form a big droplet which can easily be sucked up using a syringe
- Pour contents of the syringe into the plastic container with 5 to 10 ml of water
- Put scotch tape, if used, in the plastic container
- Put the used syringe in a separate plastic container for future use.

Storage and Disposal of Waste Mercury

The container should be stored in a central area easily accessible to healthcare worker for future spills.[58]

Scrap Amalgam

Both metals in amalgam, i.e. mercury and silver are toxic and hence detrimental to the environment and health when released. Prevent these wastes from entering the regular garbage. Municipal Corporation should enforce some laws to place concentration limits on these and other heavy metals that can enter the waste water stream. Dentists should use this material judiciously and minimize the amount that enters the environment through their waste streams.

a. Noncontact/Unused Scrap Amalgam (Fig. 11.4)

Amalgam scraps or remnants must be handled as a hazardous waste because of high mercury and silver content.

Best Management Practice (BMP)

- Separate noncontact (unused scrap) amalgam from used amalgam
- Collect it in a break resistant and airtight container.
- Label the container as "Hazardous Waste: Noncontact Scrap Amalgam"
- Once it is filled, contact a certified waste carrier for recycling or disposal.

Cautions

- Do not pour scrap amalgam particles down the drain
- Do not throw scrap amalgam into the regular garbage
- Do not mix noncontact scrap amalgam wastes with sharps wastes
- Do not handover scrap amalgam to a noncertified scrap metal dealer, unauthorized to transport hazardous wastes.[10,61]

b. Contact/Used Scrap Amalgam (Fig. 11.5).

Best Management Practice (BMP)

For Traps

Contact amalgam scrap can be managed by efficient use of traps and filters in dental office vacuum system. Disposable chair-side traps are preferred over reusable traps because amalgam particles from the trap cannot be effectively removed without spilling them into the drain or garbage. In addition, use finer traps, e.g. 100 mesh traps, as these can traps amalgam particles more effectively.

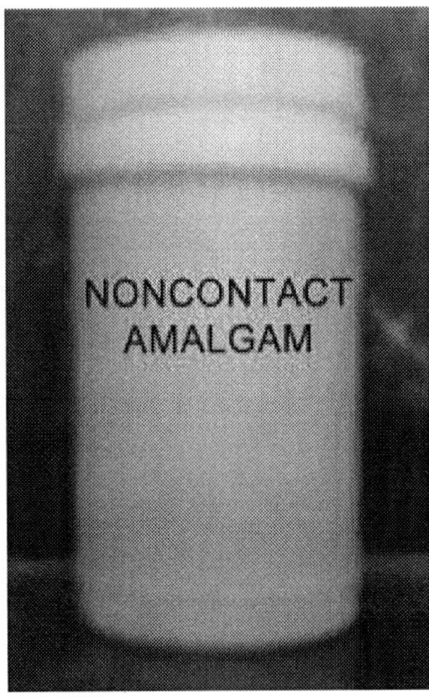

Fig. 11.4: Container for noncontact amalgam

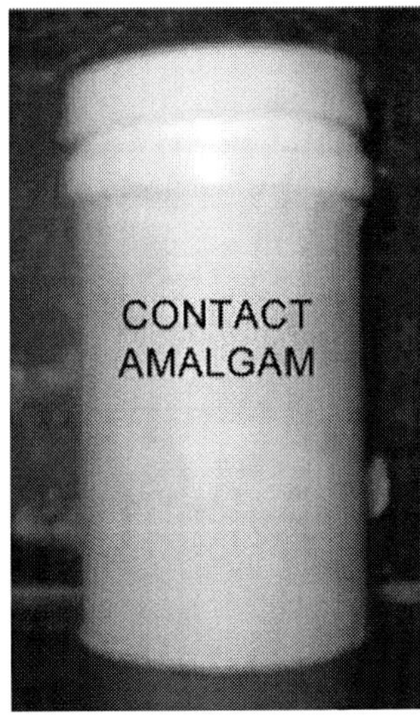

Fig. 11.5: Container for contact amalgam

However, these require strong suction system and more frequent cleaning and changing.[60]

- Flush the vacuum system with disinfecting line solution that causes minimal dissolution of amalgam (i.e. cleaners that do not contain chlorine or bleach).

A few examples of line cleansers do not contain bleach or chlorine and do not dissolve mercury from amalgam (American Dental Association):

- Biocide (Biotrol International)
- BirexSe (Biotrol International)
- Microstat 2 (Septodont USA)
- ProE-Vac (Cottrell Ltd.)
- SRG Evacuation (Icon Labs)
- Stay Clean (Apollo Dental Products)
- Turbo-Vac (Pinnacle Products)
- Vacusol Ultra (Biotrol International)
- Cavicide (Metrex Research Corp.)
- Vacuum Clean (Palmero Healthcare)
- Check with your equipment manufacturer to determine the appropriate line cleanser for your equipment*
- Remove the chair-side trap from your dental unit using universal precautions (gloves, eyewear and mask)
- Place the entire trap and its contents into a break resistant and airtight container
- Close the lid tightly
- Label the container as "Hazardous Waste: Contact scrap amalgam"[10]
- Always ask dental amalgam recycler if he will accept disposable chair-side traps in the same container with contact amalgam
- The best method is to flush the line with an appropriate line cleanser at the end of the day. The trap should be changed the next morning before the suction is used. This method will allow the particles in the trap to dry.[60]

For Vacuum Pump Filters

- Replace vacuum pump filters following manufacturer's instructions
- Use standard precautions and PPE while handling the filters
- Remove the filter and hold it over a tray or other container that can catch spills. Close the lid securely on to the filter and place it in the contact amalgam container
- Label the container as "Hazardous Waste: Contact scrap amalgam"
- When the container is filled, send for recycling
- Always make sure that amalgam recycler is certified to transport hazardous wastes and will take these filters
- Do not discard used vacuum pump filters as medical waste
- Close the lid securely on to the filter.[61]

Amalgam must be disinfected before shipment to the recycler. Do not use an autoclave or any other method that utilizes heat as heat may cause the mercury to volatilize and be released to the environment.[60]

Other Options

- For visibly clean traps and filters: Disposable ones can be thrown into the regular garbage, if reusable traps and filters can be inserted back into dental unit
- If the trap and filter are not visibly clean, treat them as hazardous wastes and place in a contact amalgam container.

Cautions

- Do not mix contact and noncontact amalgam
- Do not mix contact scrap amalgam with biomedical wastes or sharps
- Do not rinse traps and filters down the drain as amalgam particles will be discharged into the sewer
- Do not throw disposable traps containing amalgam particles into the regular garbage
- Do not wipe traps/filters with cotton, gauge or paper napkin or any other material as this creates another contaminated waste.

Note

- Traps and filters should be emptied according to the manufacturer's instructions
- Follow your manufacturer's instructions regarding equipment maintenance
- Follow the requirements of your amalgam recycler for the storage, disinfection and shipping of scrap amalgam.[10]

If you store dental amalgam scrap under water, or other liquid, do not discharge the liquid into the municipal sanitary sewer under any circumstances.[60]

Always

- Use chair-side amalgam traps and change filters regularly
- Collect scrap amalgam for recycling
- Train the staff in proper mercury/amalgam spill containment and management procedures.

Never

- Put amalgam in the sharps container
- Put amalgam scrap in the yellow biohazard or medical waste bag
- Put amalgam scrap in the trash
- Place scrap amalgam down the drain
- Use a vacuum cleaner to clean-up spilled mercury
- Rinse out chair-side traps.

Empty Amalgam Capsules

Best Management Practice

They can safely be discarded into trash.

Amalgam Separators

Amalgam separators can remove amalgam from the dental waste water more effectively than filters and traps used in chair-side dental units and vacuum lines as these can capture very fine particles.

Plumbing Replacement and Repairs

- While removing or cleaning the plumbing parts, avoid spilling the contents in case amalgam or mercury is present
- Pour and brush out the sludge and handle it in the same way as contact amalgam. Alternatively, discard it as hazardous waste
- The plumbing parts can then be reassembled or recycled.[61]

Additional sources of mercury in dental offices

- Sphygmomanometers—Content of elemental mercury in a wall-mounted sphygmomanometer is approximately 90 gm
- Thermometers—Clinical thermometers contain approximately 1 gm of mercury while it is up to 10 gm in laboratory thermometers. Digital substitutes should be preferred over mercury containing equipment
- Mercury content in fluorescent lamps ranges from 3 to 30 mg. So 'low mercury lamps' having 3 to 6 mg of mercury should be purchased. Fluorescent lamps should be collected for recycling.

Mercury-free Purchasing

Nowadays, digital sphygmomanometers, thermometers, thermostats, switches, etc. are available (Figs 11.6 and 11.7). As an alternative for fluorescent lamps, low-mercury or green-tip bulbs are available in the market. These alternative equipments should be preferred over the conventional ones.

For Economical Recycling of Mercury

Always

- Label the waste and keep meticulous records of its use and disposal
- Be aware of national and state requirements for labeling, storage and transportation
- Work with a reputed and certified medical waste hauler.[94]

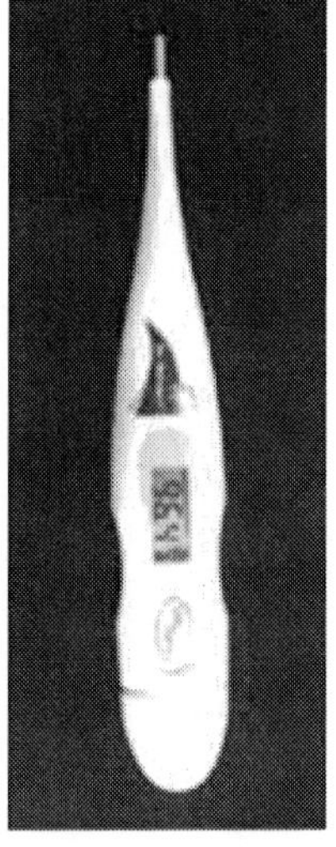

Fig. 11.6: Digital thermometer

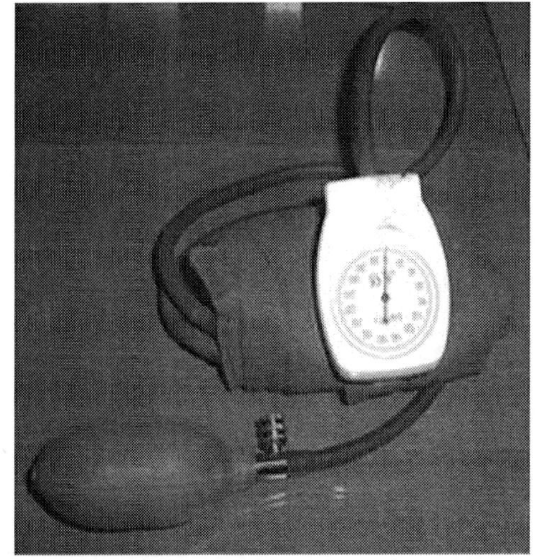

Fig. 11.7: Mercury-free sphygmomanometer

SILVER CONTAINING WASTES

Spent X-ray Fixer

Disposal Options

As spent fixer solution contains silver (a toxic substance), it contributes to the heavy metal burden in waste water. Municipal corporation can place concentration limits on several heavy metals entering the waste water stream. Dentists should also ensure that minimum amount of silver enters their waste streams (sewage system or garbage).

Best Management Practice (BMP)

- Do not mix fixer and developer solutions. In automatic processing devices, an adapter kit helps to keep these chemicals separate
- Spent fixer solution should be collected in a labeled container recommended or provided by your disposal company

- Once full, contact a certified waste carrier for recycling or disposal
- Discharge developer solution to the sewer
- Use a silver recovery unit to reclaim silver from the fixer solution and mix desilvered fixer with developer and discharge to the sewer[10]
- Utilize a digital X-ray unit, e.g. Radiovisiography (RVG), Xeroradiography to minimize the need for fixer solutions.[94]

Cautions

- Do not discharge fixer solution down the drain
- Do not throw silver recovery cartridge in the regular garbage
- Do not discharge chromium—containing cleaners into a sewer or septic system.[10]

Recycling X-ray Fixer Solution/Silver Recovery

Used fixer is the solution left over after processing X-ray films. Spent fixer solution contains very high amount of silver depending upon number and type of films processed and amount of fresh solution added to increase its strength. Therefore, silver recovery from the fixer solution is recommended. This highly concentrated silver solution (if it contains 5 mg per liter (mg/l) or more of silver) is considered as hazardous waste.

There are various recovery units/processes available for recycling of used fixer:

- **Crossover/squeegees:** They improve silver recovery by reducing carryover, i.e. the silver is kept in the fixer tank only instead of lost in the wash tank.
- **Electrolytic silver recovery:** This process uses two electrodes immersed in the fixer current. Silver ions deposit onto the cathode and thiosulfate is oxidized at the anode. Up to 95 percent of the potentially available silver can be recovered by this method, if properly operated.
- **In-line silver recovery unit:** This is an electrolytic unit through which the fixer solution is recirculated and constantly delivered in the processor tank. This results in lower silver concentration in the fixer tank 1 ounce/gal to .01 ounce/gal.

- **Metallic replacement cartridge:** This method utilizes an oxidation-reduction reaction involving elemental iron and silver thiosulfate to form ferrous iron and metallic silver. The spent fixer solution is poured into a container made up of plastic. The container can be of stainless steel, but must be lined with plastic on inner side and none of the fittings should be metallic. This container is then filled with steelwool or other metal. When the silver containing solution flows through the cartridge and contacts the steel wool, iron is released into the solution as an ion and the metallic silver is deposited on the steel wool or is released as a solid at the bottom of the cartridge and can be collected as sludge.
- **Chemical precipitation:** By adding sodium sulfide, sodium borohydride or sodium dithionite, virtually 100 percent of silver and most other metals from photographic effluent can be removed. The process results in residual silver levels of 0.5 to 1.0 mg/l.
- **Ion exchange:** This process involves removal of the silver ion from solution and its replacement with a nonsilver ion.
- **Evaporation:** This method can be used in areas not connected to any sewage system. The waste water is collected and heated to evaporate all liquids. The resulting sludge is collected in filter bags which can be sent to a silver reclaimer for recovery. It achieves "zero" water discharge.

Disadvantages of Evaporation

1. The organics and ammonia in the waste solution may also be evaporated, causing air pollution. A charcoal air filter may be used to capture the organics.
2. Filter purchase, disposal and electrical power add to operating costs.

   Never discharge liquid from which silver recovery has been done, into a septic system. Instead, it should be handled as hazardous waste.[94]

X-ray Developer

X-ray developer solution is alkaline in nature with pH 10 to 11.5.[80] If your municipality permits, it can be safely discharged to the sewer.

- Never mix X-ray developer and spent X-ray fixer because the silver containing spent X-ray fixer is a hazardous waste.
- If X-ray developer is accidentally mixed with used X-ray fixer, it must be handled as hazardous waste.

X-ray Film (Fig. 11.8)

Most of the silver content of X-ray film is removed during the processing of the film. So only traces of silver are present in a developed X-ray film and it can be discarded into the trash.

- Return unused and expired X-ray films to the manufacturer.

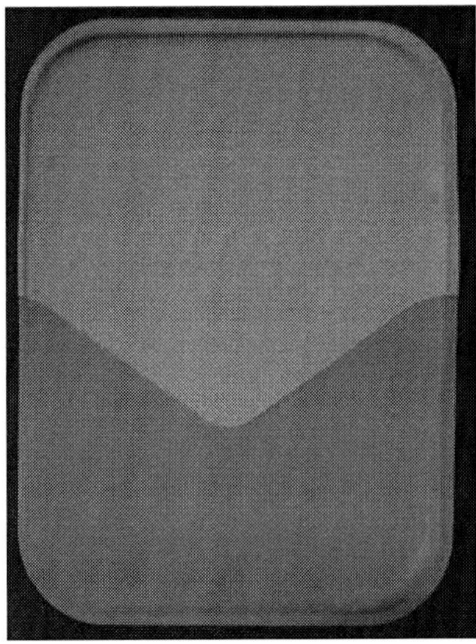

Fig. 11.8: X-ray film

Cleaners for X-ray Developer Systems

Chromium in a number of routinely used developer cleaners makes it hazardous. So carefully read the packaging label or Material Safety Data Sheet for presence of chromium. Alternatively.

- Switch to nonchromium cleaner
- Switch to digital X-ray where cleaner is not required at all.

Never put a cleaning solution and disinfectant down the drain into a septic system, regardless of its concentration. It may interfere with the proper functioning of the septic system.[94]

Developed Film (Figs 11.9A and B)

Disposal Options

Developed films are considered nonhazardous because of only traces of silver, it can be safely discarded into trash.

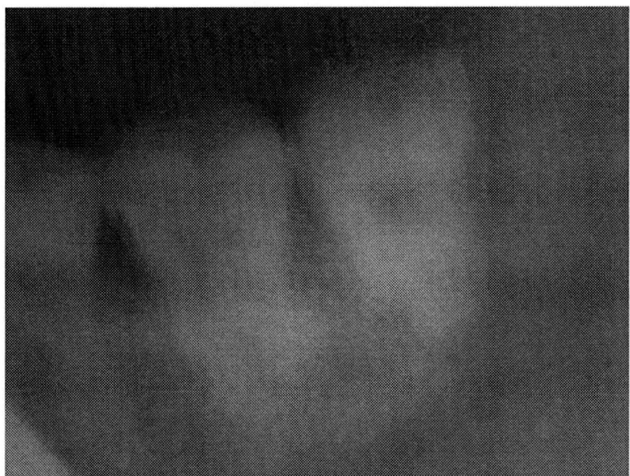

Fig. 11.9A: Developed IOPA X-ray film

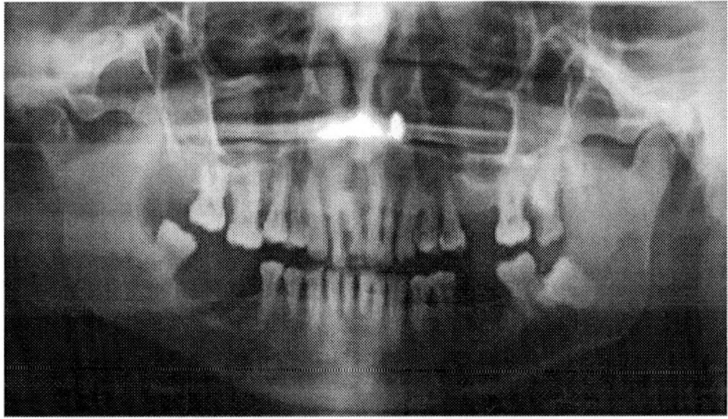

Fig.11.9B: Developed orthopantomograph

Undeveloped Film

Disposal Options

Because undeveloped film contains a high level of silver, it must be treated as a hazardous waste. Silver if sent to landfill can contaminate the soil and groundwater as it is a leachate toxin. Dentists should try to minimize the entry of silver into waste stream and recycle the unused films, if any.

Best Management Practice (BMP)

- Collect undeveloped films in a labeled container recommended or provided by your disposal company/supplier
- Send the collected films for recycling or disposal through a certified waste carrier only[10]
- Switch to digital radiography unit to minimize requirement of new X-ray films.

Advanced Radiography

Digital radiographs or computer based dental X-ray systems such as RVG, Xeroradiography, etc. require lesser (sometimes even less than 80 percent of conventional X-ray machines). Also they do not need conventional developing and fixing of exposed films as they use reusable charged instead of X-ray films. The image is processed very fast (in seconds) on a computer monitor. Also the images with minimal distortion are produced that are sharper than original X-rays. The disadvantage is that purchase of new digital equipment is a costly affair till now.[94]

Caution

Never discard undeveloped film into the regular garbage.[10]

LEAD CONTAINING WASTES

Lead foil (Fig. 11.10) packed within the X-ray film packet, protective lead shields and lead aprons should never be thrown into the trash or into biohazard bags. Instead, these can be recycled for their scrap metal content. If these lead-containing cannot be recycled, discard them as hazardous waste.

- Collect lead foils in a container and contact a certified scrap metal recycler for recycling. Many amalgam recycling agencies

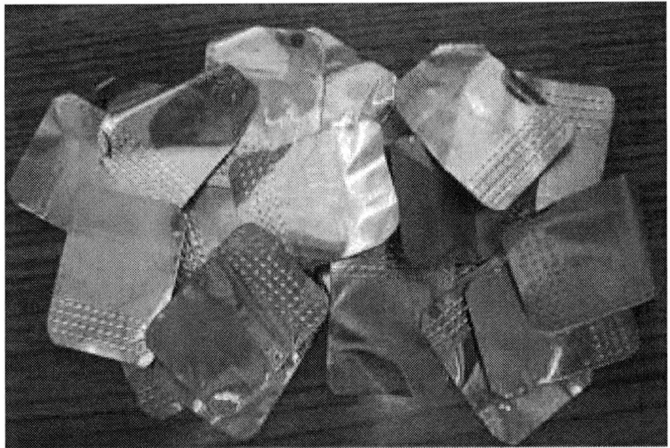

Fig. 11.10: Lead foils

and biomedical waste disposal companies also accept lead foils. Kodak also runs a recycling program for radiographic lead foils

- Always purchase durable and long-lasting lead foils, shields and aprons. Ask the suppliers if they will "take-back" the used materials and exchange them with new products
- Always double-check and have a written proof from your disposal company that hazardous wastes are being appropriately disposed.[94]

Lead Foil Packets

Best Management Practice (BMP)

Ask your film manufacturer if any recycling program is being run.

Cautions

- Do not throw lead foil packets into the general or non-hazardous waste
- Do not reuse lead foil packets for any other purpose
- Do not handover lead foil packets to your patients as they can throw them into regular garbage or can use for other purposes.

Lead Aprons

Disposal Options

Lead is a leachate toxin. If it reaches landfill sites, it can contaminate soil and groundwater. Discarded lead aprons should not be thrown in the regular garbage. Rather, dentists must contact certified waste carriers for transportation and disposal of this waste.

Best Management Practice (BMP)

Get these lead aprons recycled or disposed through a certified waste carrier.

BIOMEDICAL WASTES

Dental offices produce a number of biomedical wastes including sharps, blood soaked materials and human tissue.

Dentists must observe the liquid content of their garbage. It is the best option to mix any saliva soaked materials with other non-liquid types of garbage, (e.g. paper napkins, cotton, gloves, etc.). By doing so, dentists can avoid refusal from the landfill site.

Disposal Options

Biomedical waste must be disposed of in color-coded containers marked with the universal biohazard symbol. A number of occupational health and safety concerns related to biomedical wastes are raised for personnel handling such wastes. Therefore it is the duty of the dentists to ensure safe handling and disposal of biomedical wastes.

Anatomical Wastes (Human Tissue)

Best Management Practice (BMP)

- Keep human tissue separate from sharps and blood soaked material
- Collect it in yellow bag that is marked with the universal biohazard symbol

- There should be a locked, enclosed, designated storage area, clearly marked as a "Biomedical waste storage area", separate from other supply rooms. If storage time is expected to exceed 4 days, refrigeration at temperature $\leq 4°C$ is recommended. The universal biohazard symbol must be displayed outside
- Once sufficient waste is accumulated, contact a certified biomedical waste carrier for disposal.

Caution

Never throw human tissue into the regular garbage.

Nonanatomical Wastes (Blood Soaked Materials)

Best Management Practice (BMP)

- Do not mix blood soaked materials with sharps and other biomedical wastes
- Collect them in yellow bag
- Label the bag with a biohazard symbol
- Storage conditions remain the same as for anatomical waste
- Once sufficient waste is accumulated in the storage area, contact a certified biomedical waste carrier for disposal
- Put the wastes in double bag if quantity of liquid in the waste is high.

Items saturated with blood or body fluids, even if they are not dried or fully absorbed, must be treated as biomedical waste.

Teeth without amalgam may be thrown in regular garbage. They can also be given back to your patients after cleaning if they demand so.

Caution

Never throw blood soaked materials into the regular garbage.[10,61]

Sharps

The various types of sharps to be thrown in a sharps container are:

1. Used/unused discarded hypodermic needles, suture needles, syringes, scalpel blades, lancets and dental scalers.
2. Glass blood vials, glass culture dishes, infected Pasteur, needles with attached tubing; anesthetic carpules.

However, teeth containing amalgam are considered as hazardous wastes and should be placed in your 'contact amalgam container' and recycled through an amalgam recycler. Never put teeth containing amalgam in the yellow bag because yellow bag wastes are incinerated and the mercury in the amalgam will be volatized. Disinfect the teeth with amalgam by storing them in a container of glutaraldehyde or 10 percent formalin.[94]

Nonanatomical Wastes (Sharps, Needles, Scalpels, etc.)

Best Management Practice (BMP)

- Collect in a blue/white, rigid, puncture resistant labeled container provided by your waste carrier. The container must be a closed one with a lid that cannot be tampered with
- Put universal biohazard symbol on the container
- Once the container is three-fourth filled, contact a certified biomedical waste carrier for disposal.

Cautions

- Never throw sharps in the regular garbage
- Do not mix biomedical or other hazardous wastes with sharps waste
- Do not fill sharps container more than three-quarters full
- Do not place sharps at the curbside with your regular garbage even if your municipality accepts sterilized sharps at the landfill. Because it would create a health and safety problem for your neighborhood if per chance an animal or child gains access to your garbage.

CHEMICALS, DISINFECTANTS AND STERILIZING AGENTS

Disposal Options

A variety of chemicals are used in dental offices for sterilization, disinfection and cleaning purposes. Some of these chemicals are explosive in nature. Large volumes of such chemicals in sewage can lead to explosion. Some of the chemicals can corrode the sewage pipes with time. Before discharging any chemicals to the sewer system, contact your municipality's Public Works Department (Sewers). As the waste water gets mixed with the natural water resources eventually, it is supplied as domestic water supply. So we need to be careful.

Best Management Practice (BMP)

- Thoroughly and carefully read and follow the Material Safety Data Sheets (MSDS) for all chemicals, disinfectants and sterilizing agents used in your office
- Always get prior permission from your municipal sewers department for disposal of following chemicals to the sewer:
  - For chemicals with a flashpoint <61°C
  - For chemicals having pH $\leq$ 2.0 or pH $\geq$ 12.5
  - For chemicals containing a high concentration of formaldehyde.

Except the above-mentioned chemicals, all other chemicals, disinfectants and sterilizing agents can be safely discharged into the sewer. It is recommended to mix them with a large volume of water or flush the drain well while disposing them off.

- The empty containers can be recycled through your local recycle program or it can be discarded into the trash after rinsing it thoroughly.

Cautions

- Do not discharge inflammable substances (straight alcohols, ether, chloroform, acetone, and xylol) or other solvents down the drain without contacting your municipality first
- Do not discharge X-ray cleaning solutions containing chromium down the drain
- Do not discharge any used or unused chemicals containing high concentrations of formaldehyde, down the drain without contacting your municipality first.[10]

Autoclaves/Chemiclaves

- Spent chemiclave solution is the left over liquid after chemical sterilization of dental instruments. This solution is an ignitable waste as it contains approximately 25 percent alcohol and has a flash-point below 140°F

- Neither discharge chemiclave solution to the municipal sanitary sewer nor discard into the trash because it is ignitable. Instead, discard it as hazardous waste.

Drugs and Pharmaceutical Chemicals

Never throw unused or used drugs (Fig. 11.11) and pharmaceutical chemicals in the general waste. Many of the commonly used drugs are actually hazardous such as iodine, alcohol, silver nitrate, methanol, mercuric oxide, etc. Mercury is a component of many vaccines and laboratory uses. Furthermore, certain commonly used pharmaceuticals such as epinephrine, nicotine patches and warfarin are considered to be "acutely hazardous" and require additional handling requirements if a certain concentration limit is exceeded.

"Nonhazardous" drugs should also not be thrown in the trash because of liability issues. A plan must be developed for segregating and managing the unused drugs and pharmaceutical chemicals.

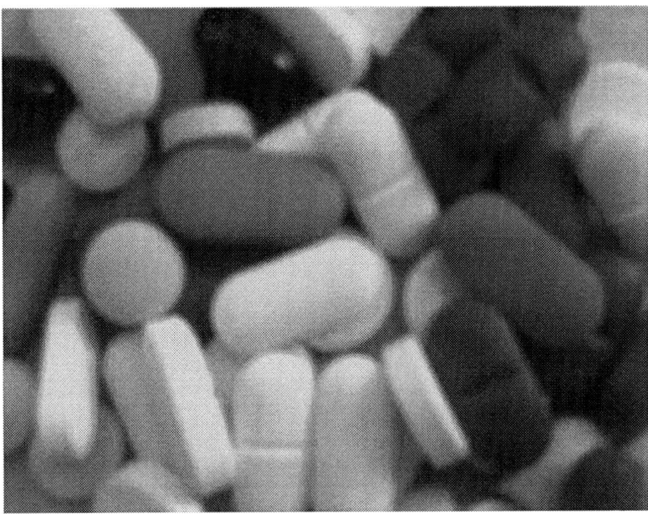

Fig. 11.11: Pharmaceutical waste

- Segregate the unused drugs from other trash. Unless you are certain about a particular drug that it is not a hazardous waste, assume it to be hazardous and discard it appropriately through a licensed hazardous waste hauler
- Never pour discarded drugs down the drain if your office is on a septic field
- Ask your pharmaceutical distributor to take back unused or expired drugs and for help in designating particular drugs
- Do not accept drug samples unless you are sure that you can use them or return them
- Do not put unused drugs in the red bag wastes because most red bag wastes are treated through steam-sterilization.[94]

Some Other Dental Wastes

1. **Office waste:** As most of the office waste is usually not hazardous, it goes to the regular garbage. However aluminum, glass, paper (including cardboard, newspaper, etc.) should be recycled. Many garbage haulers or recycling centers have their system for collection of such wastes.
2. **Computer waste:** The cathode ray tubes used in monitors and televisions contain 5 to 8 lbs of lead in the tube. Computer components also contain heavy metals (e.g. Mercury) and other materials like plastics. Many of these materials are not easily recycled. Till a few years ago, computers were often disposed at the landfills or in the incinerator. At the landfill sites, they diminish valuable landfill capacity and release leachate toxins into the soil and ground water. If incinerated, toxic emissions into the environment are released.

Best Management Practice (BMP)

1. Instead of purchasing new ones, upgrade and reuse perfectly good parts.
2. Review your electronics vendor. You should know and approve of the final destination of these materials.
3. Do not break cathode ray tubes to reduce volume.[60]

POLLUTION PREVENTION FOR DENTISTS

Dentists should incorporate pollution prevention activities into their practices so as to minimize the amount of hazardous materials requiring disposal. Wherever feasible, dental offices should replace/substitute hazardous substances with less toxic or nontoxic ones. Examples include:

- Use precapsulated amalgams instead of liquid (elemental) mercury. These are available in a wide range of sizes. Hence, it becomes easier to minimize scrap amalgam by selecting the appropriate size for individual restoration
- Stay updated with advances in restorative materials and provides patients with complete information about the associated benefits and risks
- Do not purchase excessive quantity of chemicals, disinfectants and sterilants to avoid disposal of excess
- To clean X-ray equipment, use soap and water only
- Do not purchase inflammable chemicals, i.e. those with a flashpoint below 61°C
- Switch to digital radiography.[10]

A quick review of dental waste management is given below (Table 11.1):

Table 11.1: A quick review of dental waste management mercury/amalgam waste handling procedures

Type of waste	*Generating procedure*	*Management*	*Caution*
Extracted teeth with amalgam	Dental extractions	1. Use universal precautions when handling extracted teeth 2. Place in the contact amalgam container 3. Recycle through an amalgam recycler.	**DO NOT:** 1. Place in the biohazard bag 2. Place in the trash 3. Place in the sharps container.
Elemental mercury	Bulk mercury containers,spills and spill clean-up	1. Always wear nitrile gloves when cleaning up a spill 2. Train staff in spill clean-up procedures 3. Recycle unused bulk mercury through a recycler.	**DO NOT:** 1. Discharge to municipal sanitary sewer 2. Place in the trash 3. Place in the biohazard bag 4. Place in the sharps container 5. Clean-up spills with a vacuum cleaner.
Empty amalgam capsules	Fillings, restoration work	1. Discard into the trash.	
Broken or unusable amalgam capsules	Fillings, restoration work	1. Collect and store contents with scrap amalgam for recycling.	**DO NOT:** 1. Place in the trash 2. Place in the biohazard bag 3. Place in the sharps container.
Scrap amalgam	Traps, screens, excess mix, vacuum pump filters	1. Store in labeled containers 2. Send to a recycler 3. Recycle heavily contaminated traps.	**DO NOT:** 1. Place in the biohazard bag 2. Discharge to municipal sanitary sewer

Contd...

Contd...

Type of waste	*Generating procedure*	*Management*	*Caution*
		4. Recycle vacuum pump filters.	3. Place in the sharps container 4. Place in the trash 5. Disinfect with any method that uses heat.
Broken thermo-meters and blood pressure units	Accidental breakage	1. Clean-up visible mercury with mercury spill kit—always wear nitrile gloves 2. Place contaminated items in container that will not leak or rupture; label as required by law 3. Discard contaminated items through a hazardous waste hauler	**DO NOT:** 1. Place contaminated items in the trash 2. Place contaminated items in the biohazard bag. 3. Place contaminated items in the sharps container.
Biomedical waste	Dental treatment	Sharps: Discard as biomedical waste in sharp container Blood and body fluids: Discard as biomedical waste a. **If** less than 20 cubic cm discharge to the municipal sanitary sewer. b. **If** more than 20 cubic cm discard as biomedical waste	**DO NOT:** 1. Mix with hazardous waste 2. Mix with amalgam.

Contd...

Contd...

Type of waste	*Generating procedure*	*Management*	*Caution*
		Contact wastes (gloves, aprons): a. Teeth without amalgam: Disinfect with glutaraldehyde or 10% formalin, then may be given to patient or place in trash. b. Teeth with amalgam: Disinfect with glutaraldehyde or 10% formalin then put in contact amalgam container.	
Unused pharmaceutical chemicals	Dental treatment	1. Return to manufacturer 2. Discard as hazardous waste.	**DO NOT:** 1. Place in the trash 2. Discharge into the municipal sanitary sewer.
Radiographic films	Processing of radiograph	a. Processed films: Discard in trash b. Unprocessed films: Send for recycling.	**DO NOT:** 1. Discharge used X-ray fixer into the municipal sanitary sewer.
Used X-ray developer solution	Processing of radiograph	1. Can be discharged to local municipal sanitary sewer	1. **DO NOT** mix X-ray developer and used X-ray fixer. 2. If mixing occurs, discard mixture as hazardous waste
Used X-ray fixer solution	Processing of radiograph	a. Discard as hazardous waste. OR Send to silver reclamation facility b. Buy your personal silver recovery unit.	

Contd...

Contd...

Type of waste	*Generating procedure*	*Management*	*Caution*
Chromium-containing X-ray system cleaners	Cleaning of X-ray system	1. Discard as hazardous waste 2. Switch to nonchromium cleaners	1. **DO NOT** discharge cleaners containing chromium into the municipal sanitary sewer
Lead foils and shields	X-ray processing, protective shields	1. Foil: Recycle through a scrap metal dealer or discard as hazardous waste 2. Shields/aprons: Return the worn out shields/aprons to the manufacturer and replace with a new one	**DO NOT:** 1. Place in the trash 2. Place in the biohazard bag
Chemiclave/ Chemical sterilant solutions	Sterilization of dental instruments	Discard as hazardous waste	**DO NOT:** 1. Discharge chemiclave solution to the municipal sanitary sewer 2. Flush down septic system
Disinfectants and cleaners	General office cleaning	Follow the instructions written on the label for handling and disposal	DO NOT discharge to municipal sanitary sewer
Alcohols, ethers, peroxides		Discard as hazardous waste	DO NOT discharge to municipal sanitary sewer
Glutaraldehyde	Disinfection of dental instruments	Diluted glutaraldehyde may be discharged to the municipal sanitary sewer	**DO NOT** flush down septic system
Office waste	General fluorescent bulbs and ballasts batteries	Recycle all fluorescent bulbs and ballasts battery	**DO NOT:** 1. Place in trash 2. Place in the trash, biohazard bag, or sharps container

Source: *The environmentally responsible dental office: A guide to proper waste management in Connecticut dental office. Northeast natural resource center of the national wildlife federation and state of Connecticut, department of environmental protection; 2000.*

CHAPTER

12 Training of Healthcare Workers

Infectious healthcare waste increases the risk of nosocomial infections and puts the health of medical staff and the patients at risk. So appropriate measures should be taken for systematic and precise handling, treatment/disposal of healthcare waste. A policy for the management of heathcare waste cannot be effective unless it is implemented carefully, consistently and universally.[66]

Training of healthcare workers is the core of healthcare waste management programs. Regular training and workshops of the workers should therefore be conducted.

- Each and every healthcare establishment must have well-planned awareness and training program in place for all categories of personnel including administrators (medical, paramedical and administrative)
- All the healthcare professionals must be made aware of Bio-medical Waste (Management and Handling) Rules, 1998 and subsequent amendments
- Healthcare establishment should introduce awards for safe healthcare waste management and universal precaution practices
- Training should be imparted to all categories of personnel in appropriate language/medium and in an acceptable manner.[20]

The training should be continuous, comprehensive, integrated and structured with the necessary elements.[48]

AIMS OF TRAINING

The aim of training of biomedical waste handlers is to develop awareness about the safety, health and environmental issues related to healthcare waste and their effect on workers in their daily work. Public health and safety at work place and environmental awareness are responsibility of all and in the interest of all.[66]

The focus of training program should be on the local legislative controls, so as to deal with:

- Waste matter
- Practical measures available for waste minimization
- Techniques for better management of resources

Specifically the training program should focus on:

- Recent and updated guidelines for segregation, management and disposal of infectious or potentially infectious healthcare waste
- Providing the guidelines to the healthcare system on the opportunities for waste minimization and the reduction of air pollution from incineration of biomedical waste
- Various strategies and appropriate techniques for handling of biomedical waste management
- Minimizing the incidence of spread of disease to healthcare worker and the public due to a disease or injury contracted from healthcare waste
- Creating awareness about hospital accreditation with focus on guidelines about healthcare safety issues related with disposal of BMW
- Understanding the new technologies available for safe disposal of biomedical waste with eco-friendly approach and infection control in healthcare establishments.[97]

WHO NEEDS TRAINING?

Four main categories of personnel should be kept in mind while planning training activities:

1. Hospital management members and administrative staff because they are responsible for implementing regulations on healthcare waste management.
2. Medical doctors, dental surgeons.
3. Nurses, assistant nurses and laboratory personnel.
4. Auxiliary staff, cleaners, transporters, and waste handlers.

Management of the healthcare establishment should make strategies for training of personnel at all the levels. The administrators should design separate courses for the categories listed above. These strategies should be adapted specifically to their tasks, responsibilities and level of education.

Hands on training should be provided wherever appropriate. Testing the participants at the end of the course, by means of simple true/false or objective type questions allows the course organizers to make assessment about the knowledge acquired by participants and provides an incentive for learning. Courses should be repeated periodically to refresh and update training as well as orientation for new employees and for existing employees with new responsibilities; it will also help update knowledge in line with policy changes.

Responsibility for all training related to the segregation, collection, storage and disposal of healthcare waste should be given to the ICO (Infection Control Officer). It is his/her responsibility to ensure that staff at all levels are well aware both of the hospital waste management plan and policy, and of their own responsibilities and obligations.

A training protocol could be developed by the national government agency/international agency responsible for the disposal of healthcare wastes. Drawings, diagrams, photographs, slides or overhead transparencies should be maximally used. These should represent the conditions in which trainees work and suggest examples of measures that have been (or will be) implemented. It is likely that waste handlers and other workers are illiterate; so to help them understand all procedures should be carefully illustrated in diagrams and photographs.

Selection of Participants

The ideal number of participants in a training course is twenty to thirty. All categories of personnel should be targeted. Groups composed of trainers from different levels may make the discussion easier and more useful, as one can make others understand the points which are difficult for them.

RECOMMENDATIONS FOR TRAINING OF HEALTH-CARE PERSONNEL

Training course must put emphasis on the following points:

1. Never mix hazardous and general waste. If the two are mixed accidentally, the entire mixture should be treated as hazardous healthcare waste.
2. Correction of segregation mistakes by removing items from a bag or container or by placing one bag into another of a different color should not be attempted in any case.
3. Nursing and clinical staff should ensure that bag holders and containers for the collection, and subsequent on-site storage of healthcare waste in the wards, clinics, and operation theaters are provided in adequate number. These containers should be placed as close to the common sources of waste as is possible.
4. The greatest care should be taken while removing needles from syringes.

RECOMMENDATIONS FOR TRAINING OF WASTE HANDLERS

It is observed that the routine healthcare waste handlers tend to become less precise/particular about safety measures. This can increase the risk of injury. Therefore, periodic refresher training is recommended. Points that should be emphasized upon in the training of waste handlers are:

- Adequate protective clothing should be worn during handling of healthcare waste
- Do not mix bags for hazardous healthcare waste with those for general waste. Instead keep them segregated throughout handling; hazardous waste should be placed only in specified storage areas
- Check that waste storage bags and containers are sealed. Bags should not be removed unless they are properly labeled and securely sealed to prevent spillages
- Avoid contact of body with the waste bags during handling. Collectors should not carry too many bags at a time (not more than two)

- Always pick the bags up by the neck only. However, minimize manual handling of waste bags whenever possible
- Do not throw or drop the waste bags to avoid puncture or other damage
- Sharps may occasionally puncture the side or bottom of a polypropylene container; so carry the container by its handle and do not support underneath with the free hand
- In the event of accidental spillage, follow appropriate cleaning and disinfection procedures. If a spillage occurs, report immediately to the responsible staff member.

TRAINING FOR WASTE TRANSPORTATION STAFF

Transportation of waste can be carried out by either the healthcare establishment itself or an authorized waste transporter. Drivers and waste handlers should be well aware of the nature and risks of the waste being transported. They should be able to follow the instruction to carry out all the procedures, without help from others.

Transportation staff should be trained in procedures listed below.

1. The wearing of protective clothing and strong footwear during handling.
2. Correct methods/procedures for handling, loading, and unloading of waste bags and containers.
3. Procedures for handling spillages or other accidents; written instructions for these procedures should be provided in the transport vehicle.
4. Keeping in mind any accidental spillage during loading, transport or unloading, spare plastic bags, protective clothing and the cleaning tools and disinfectants should always be available in transport vehicles.
5. Documentation and recording of healthcare waste, e.g. a consignment note system, traced from the point of collection to the final place of disposal.

Untrained personnel should never be allowed to handle hazardous healthcare waste.

TRAINING OF OPERATORS OF TREATMENT PLANTS

For incinerators and other treatment facilities, qualified operators are required. If qualified operators are unavailable, it is the responsibility of healthcare establishments to arrange for training of an adequate number of personnel. Educational qualification of treatment plant operators should be at least secondary school level plus technical education. They should be trained particularly in the following areas:

1. Health, safety, and environmental effects of treatment operations.
2. Technical procedures for operation of the plant.
3. General working of the treatment facility including heat recovery and flue-gas cleaning technologies, where appropriate.
4. Maintenance of the plant.
5. Surveillance of the quality of ash and emissions, according to the specifications.
6. In case of equipment failures, emergency responses, e.g. alarms.
7. Record-keeping.

TRAINING OF LANDFILL OPERATORS

The training of landfill operators is essential for minimizing the risks associated with buried healthcare waste, in relation to both scavenging and the quality of groundwater. Landfill operators should therefore be trained in the following issues:

1. Risks related to health due to healthcare waste.
2. Use of protective equipment and personal hygiene.
3. Hazards related to the sorting of healthcare waste, which should not be carried out either by the landfill operators or by other people.
4. Safe procedures for landfilling the wastes.
5. Minimizing the handling of healthcare waste by drivers or site operators.
6. Procedures for emergency response, in case of any accident.

PUBLIC AWARENESS ON HAZARDS OF HEALTHCARE WASTE

The objectives of public education on healthcare waste are the following:

1. To make hospital patients and visitors aware about hygiene and healthcare waste management.
2. To prevent any voluntary or accidental exposure to healthcare waste.
3. To inform about the risks associated with healthcare waste, with a focus on people living or working in close proximity to or visiting healthcare establishments, families of patients receiving treatment at home and scavengers on waste dumps.

The following measures can be taken for public education on risks, segregation of waste, or waste disposal practices:

1. **Poster exhibitions** on healthcare waste issues, including the risks involved in scavenging discarded sharps, e.g. syringes and hypodermic needles. Posters should be self-explanatory i.e. diagrams and illustrations should convey the message to masses, including illiterate people.
2. **Explanation** of waste management policy to the incoming patients and visitors, by the staff of healthcare establishments, by means of distributing leaflets.
3. All information should be displayed or communicated in an attractive manner to hold public attention.
4. In the healthcare establishment, waste bins should be easily accessible to patients and visitors. These should be clearly marked with the label of intended waste category.[66]

CHAPTER

13 Immunization of Healthcare Workers

Working in a healthcare establishment may pose various health-related challenges in the form of infections. The healthcare workers can acquire these infections either from the patients or patient-related materials. They can also transmit infections to other patients and other employees. Healthcare workers are prone to HIV, hepatitis B and C viral infections.

Employee's health status should be determined at the time of recruitment, with details of immunization history, previous exposures to communicable diseases, (e.g. tuberculosis) and immune status at present. Healthcare workers who have acquired infections should report their illnesses/incident to staff incharge for further evaluation and management. Thus, an employee's health program must be in place to prevent and manage infections in hospital staff. Immunization recommended for staff includes: hepatitis A and B, influenza, measles, mumps, rubella, tetanus, and diphtheria. Immunization against varicella, rabies may be considered in specific cases.[98]

MANAGEMENT OF OCCUPATIONAL BLOOD EXPOSURES

1st Step

Immediate Care to the Exposure Site

- Wash wounds and skin with soap and water
- Flush mucous membranes with clean water.

2nd Step

Risk Assessment

It depends upon: **Type of fluid**, e.g. blood, fluid contaminated with blood, other potentially infectious fluid or tissue, and concentrated virus.

Type of exposure: For example, percutaneous injury, mucous membrane or nonintact skin exposure, and bites or pricks resulting in blood exposure.

3rd Step

Evaluation of the Exposed Person

Assess immune status for infection (i.e. by history of hepatitis B vaccination and vaccine response).

4th Step

Postexposure Prophylaxis

It should be administered for exposures posing risk of transmission of infection. For example, infections like:
- HCV: Postexposure Prophylaxis (PEP) not recommended
- HBV
- HIV
  - PEP should be initiated at the earliest, preferably within hours of exposure.
  - Pregnancy test should be offered to all women of childbearing age who are not known to be pregnant.
  - If viral resistance is suspected, experts should be consulted.
  - PEP should be administered for four weeks if tolerated.

5th Step

Follow-up Testing and Counseling

Exposed persons must seek medical evaluation for any acute illness which occurs during follow-up.

HBV Exposures

Perform follow-up anti-HBs testing in persons who have received hepatitis B vaccine.
- The follow-up test for anti-HBs should be done 1 to 2 months after last dose of vaccine
- Anti-HBs response to vaccine cannot be ascertained if the person has received HBIG in the past 3 to 4 months.

HCV Exposures

- Baseline testing and follow-up testing for anti-HCV and Alanine aminotransferase (ALT) should be performed 4 to 6 months after exposure
- If earlier diagnosis of HCV infection is desired, perform HCV RNA at 4 to 6 weeks
- Confirm repeatedly by performing reactive anti-HCV Enzyme Immunoassays (EIAs) with supplemental tests.

HIV Exposures

- HIV-antibody testing should be performed for a minimum of 6 months postexposure (e.g. at baseline, 6 weeks, 3 months, and 6 months).
- HIV antibody testing should be performed if illness similar to/associated with an acute retroviral syndrome occurs.
- Exposed persons must be advised to use precautions and preventive barriers to prevent secondary transmission of HIV during the follow-up period.
- Exposed persons taking PEP should be evaluated within 72 hours after exposure.
- Exposed persons taking PEP should be monitored for drug toxicity for a minimum of 2 weeks.[93]

Tetanus and Diphtheria Vaccination

This can be done according to the person's history of primary vaccination series with tetanus toxoid-containing vaccine.

1. *Adults with uncertain histories of a complete primary vaccination*: They should receive a primary series using combined tetanus and diphtheria toxoid as Td.
2. *Adults with history of complete primary vaccination*: They should receive one booster dose if the last vaccination was received > 10 years previously.
3. *Adults ≥ 50 years of age with complete pediatric series, plus the teenage/young adult booster*: They should receive a booster dose only.

Measles, Mumps, Rubella (MMR)

A second dose of MMR is recommended in the following cases:
1. Adults with recent exposure to measles or in an epidemic condition.
2. Adults previously vaccinated with killed measles vaccine.
3. Healthcare workers.

Rubella Component

For women of childbearing age, irrespective of age, rubella immunity should be routinely determined and women should be counselled about congenital rubella syndrome. Administer 1 dose of MMR vaccine to women with uncertain history of rubella vaccination or who lack laboratory evidence of immunity. Do not vaccinate women who are pregnant or who might become pregnant within 4 weeks of receiving vaccine. Such women should receive MMR vaccine upon completion or termination of pregnancy and before they are discharged from the healthcare facility.

Varicella Vaccination

Special consideration should be given to those who have close contact with persons at high risk for severe disease (healthcare workers).[73]

HEPATITIS A VACCINATION

Prevention of hepatitis A can be done through active or passive immunization.

Hepatitis A vaccine is available as the single-antigen vaccines havrix, vaqta and the combination vaccine Twinrix® (contains both HAV and HBV antigens). All these are inactivated vaccines.

Prophylaxis Against Hepatitis A Virus Infection

Immunoglobulin (IG) (Passive Immunization)

IG is a sterile preparation of concentrated antibodies (immunoglobulins) and is made from pooled human plasma processed by cold ethanol fractionation observed. IG protects against hepatitis A virus infection through passive transfer of antibody. IG can be administered intramuscularly (IM) and intravenously. Both IGIM and IGIV contain anti-HAV, but IG administered intramuscularly is the preferred product to be used for the prevention of HAV infection. Concentration of IgG anti-HAV achieved after administration of IG intramuscularly are below the level of detection through the majority of commercially available diagnostic tests.

- For pre-exposure prophylaxis (Tables 13.1 and 13.2)

Administration of 1 dose of 0.02 ml/kg IM provides protection for < 3 months, and 1 dose of 0.06 ml/kg IM provides protection for 3 to 5 months.

- For postexposure prophylaxis

Administration of 0.02 ml/kg IM, within 2 weeks of exposure is recommended which is 80 to 90 percent effective in preventing hepatitis A. Administration of IG requires an appropriate muscle mass (i.e. the deltoid or gluteal muscle) into which a substantial volume can be injected. For children aged < 24 months, the anterolateral thigh muscle should be chosen for IM injection.

Table 13.1: Recommended doses of immunoglobulin (IG) for hepatitis A pre-exposure and postexposure prophylaxis

Setting	*Duration of coverage*	*Dose (ml/kg)*
Pre-exposure	Short-term (1 to 2 months)	0.02
	Long-term (3 to 5 months)	0.06*
Postexposure		0.02

*Repeat every 5 months if continued exposure to hepatitis A virus occurs.

Source: *MMWR. Prevention of hepatitis A through active or passive immunization, 2006.*

Table 13.2: Recommended doses of VAQTA: Inactivated hep. A vaccine

Age of the vaccine recipient	*Dose (Units) (U)*	*Vol. (ml)*	*No. doses*	*Schedule (months)**
12 months to 18 yrs	25	0.5	2	0,6 to 18
≥ 19 yrs	50	1.0	2	0,6 to 18

*0 months represents of initial dose: Subsequent numbers represent the duration in months after the initial dose during which 2nd dose can be given any time.

Source: MMWR. Prevention of hepatitis A through active or passive immunization, 2006.

Table 13.3: Recommended doses of havrix: Inactivated hepatitis A vaccine[66]

Age of the vaccine recipient	Dose enzyme-linked immunosorbent assay units (ELU)	Vol. (ml) doses	No. of (months)	Schedule
12 months to 18 yr	720	0.5	2	0,6-12
≥ 19 yr	1440	1.0	2	0,6-12

Source: MMWR. Prevention of hepatitis A through active or passive immunization, 2006.

Table 13.4: Recommended doses of twinrix : Combine inactivated hepatitis A and hepatitis B vaccine

Age of the vaccine recipient	Dose (hepatitis A/hepatitis B) ELU*/20 µg	Vol. (ml)	No. doses	Schedule (months)
≥ 18 yr	720	1.0	3	0,1,6
≥ 18 yr	720	1.0	4	0,7,21 days + 1 yr

***ELU**—ELISA units

Source: *CDC. Travelers' Health-Yellow Book, 2009.*

Note: IG can be safely administered during pregnancy or lactation.

Hepatitis A Vaccine (Tables 13.3 and 13.4)

Twinrix

Combined inactivated hepatitis A and hepatitis B vaccine.

The dosage of the hepatitis A component in the combined vaccine is lower than that in the single-antigen hepatitis A vaccine. So it can be administered in a 3-dose schedule instead of 2-dose schedule used for the single-antigen vaccine.

Contraindications and Precautions

Hepatitis A vaccine is should not be administered in persons with a history of a severe allergic reaction to a previous dose of hepatitis A vaccine or to a vaccine component of the vaccine.

Postexposure Prophylaxis with IG

Persons, who have been vaccinated with 1 dose of hepatitis A vaccine approximately 1 month before exposure to HAV, do not need IG. However, those who have not been previously vaccinated, should be administered a single dose of IG (0.02 ml/kg) IM as soon as possible.

A reliable diagnosis of hepatitis cannot be made on clinical presentation alone, so serologic confirmation of HAV infection is must. This confirmatory serologic testing for hepatitis A virus infection should be performed by IgM anti-HAV testing of the index patients before administering postexposure treatment to contacts. It is not recommended to screen contacts for immunity before administering IG as screening would result in delay.

In a nonvaccinated person with a recent exposure to HAV infection, IG can be administered simultaneously with HA vaccine, but on a different anatomic injection site. Hepatitis A vaccine is not licensed for use as postexposure prophylaxis.[65]

HEPATITIS B VACCINE DOSE AND ADMINISTRATION (TABLES 13.5 AND 13.6)

When the 3-dose vaccine series is administered intramuscularly to healthy adults aged ≤ 40 years, with a dose schedule of 0, 1, and 6 months, a protective antibody response is produced in approximately 30 to 55 percent of individuals with first dose, 75 percent with the second dose, and > 90 percent after the third dose.

Protective antibody response declines with age. It is observed that < 90 percent individuals above 40 years, and 75 percent persons aged 60 years develop protective levels of antibody after 3-dose vaccination regimen. In addition to age, other host factors such as obesity, genetic factors, smoking and immune suppression also contribute to decreased response to vaccine. Alternative vaccination schedules, (e.g. 0, 1, and 4 months or 0, 2, and 4 months) elicit similar dose-specific and final rates of seroprotection as obtained on a 0, 1, 6 months schedule.

Hepatitis B vaccine should be administered by intramuscular injection. The deltoid muscle is the recommended site of administration for adults as injection into the buttock is less immunogenic. Intradermal administration can result in a lower seroconversion rate and final concentration of anti-HBsAg compared with intramuscular administration.

Hepatitis B vaccine and other vaccines administered simultaneously should be given in different injection sites.

Table 13.5: Recommended doses of currently licensed formulations of adult hepatitis B vaccine, by group and vaccine type

Group	*Single-antigen vaccine*				*Combination vaccine*	
	Recombivax HB		*Engerix B*		*Twinrix*	
	Dose (μg)	*Vol. (ml)*	*Dose (μg)*	*Vol. (ml)*	*Dose (μg)*	*Vol. (ml)*
Adults (aged > 20 years)	10	1.0	20	1.0	20	1.0

Dose given in μg indicates recombinant HBsAg protein dose.

Source: MMWR. A comprehensive immunization strategy to eliminate transmission of hepatitis B virus infection in the United States, 2006.

Table 13.6: Recommended doses of hepatitis B vaccine schedules for adults (aged >20 years)

0, 1, and 6 months
0, 1, and 4 months
0, 2, and 4 months
0,1, 2, and 12 months· (For Engerix B® —for all age groups)
All schedules are applicable to single-antigen hepatitis B vaccines: Twinrix (combined hepatitis A and hepatitis B vaccine) may be administered at 0, 1, and 6 months.

Source: MMWR. A comprehensive immunization strategy to eliminate transmission of hepatitis B virus infection in the United States, 2006.

Anti-HBs concentrations of ≥ 10 mIU/ml after preexposure vaccination confer almost complete protection against both acute disease and chronic infection, even if anti-HBs concentrations decline subsequently to < 10 mIU/ml.

Hepatitis B Immunoglobulin (HBIG) Dose and Administration

- The standard adult dose of HBIG is 0.06 ml/kg
- Route of administration —IM, deltoid/gluteal region
- HBIG and HB vaccine may be administered simultaneously, but in a different injection site
- A standard dose HBIG provides passively acquired anti-HBs and temporary protection, (i.e. 3–6 months). For postexposure immunoprophylaxis to prevent HBV infection, HBIG typically

is used in addition to hepatitis B vaccine. Those who do not respond to hepatitis B vaccination, HBIG is the primary means of protection after an HBV exposure.

Unknown or Uncertain Vaccination Status

Persons, whose written documentation of vaccination is not available, should be considered susceptible and age-appropriate vaccine schedule should be started or continued.

Interrupted Vaccine Schedules

- Vaccine series does not need to be restarted if the hepatitis B vaccine schedule is interrupted
- If the series is interrupted after the first dose, the second dose should be administered at the earliest; the second and third doses should be administered after a minimum of 8 weeks interval
- If only the third dose has been delayed, it should be administered as soon as possible.

Minimum Dosing Intervals and Management of Persons who were Vaccinated Inadequately

- The time gap between 2nd and 3rd dose of vaccine should not be less than 8 weeks and that between 3rd and 1st should be a minimum of 16 weeks. The minimum interval between the first and second doses is 4 weeks
- If the dose of hepatitis B vaccine was inadequate or dose interval between successive doses was shorter than recommended, the person should be revaccinated, using correct dosage or schedule.

Postvaccination Testing for Serological Response

- Serological response should be tested 1 to 2 months after administration of the last dose of the vaccine series
- If anti-HBs concentration is ≥ 10 mIU/ml—Immune.
  If anti-HBs concentration is ≤ 10 mIU/ml—Revaccinate

Revaccinated persons, who reveal inadequate protective concentration of anti-HBs, should be tested for HBsAg.

– HBsAg +ve persons — manage appropriately

- HBsAg –ve persons — they are prone to get HBV infection and should take precautionary preventive measures.

Prophylactic HBIG should be administered for any known/ unknown exposure.

Booster Doses

Previously vaccinated immunocompetent individuals do not need booster dose. However when anti-HBs levels decline to < 10 mIU/ml, a booster dose should be administered. Annual anti-HBs testing should also be considered for such cases.

Postexposure Prophylaxis to Prevent Hepatitis B Virus Infection

For HBsAg Positive Exposure Source

1. Vaccinated persons with written documents of hepatitis B vaccine series .... Single vaccine booster dose.
2. Persons undergoing vaccination .... HBIG administration and completion of vaccination series.
3. Unvaccinated individuals .... HBIG and HB vaccine (within 24 hr) at separate injection sites. Vaccination series should be completed as per age and schedule.

Exposure Source with Unknown HBsAg Status

- For persons with written documentation of a complete hepatitis B vaccine series, no further treatment is required
- Persons, who are undergoing vaccination, should complete the vaccine series
- For unvaccinated persons, hepatitis B vaccine series should be started at the earliest after exposure, with the first dose administered preferably within 24 hours.

Guidelines for postexposure prophylaxis of persons with nonoccupational exposures through blood or blood containing body fluids, or other exposure types and vaccination status are as follows:

1. *For HBsAg positive source:*
   - Unvaccinated contact persons should be administered hepatitis B vaccine series and HBIG.

- Vaccinated persons should be administered hepatitis B booster dose.

2. *For Unknown status of the exposure source*:
   - Unvaccinated contact persons should receive hepatitis B vaccination series
   - Vaccinated persons require no treatment.

In susceptible persons, postexposure immunoprophylaxis should be administered at the earliest (preferably within 24 hrs) as it is effective if given within 7 days for percutaneous exposure or within 14 days for sexual exposure. Hepatitis B vaccination must be completed as per age and schedule.

Contraindications and Precautions

Hepatitis B vaccination should not be administered to persons with a history of hypersensitivity to yeast or any component of vaccine. Hepatitis B vaccination is not contraindicated in pregnancy as the vaccine does not harm the fetus.[1]

MANAGEMENT OF OCCUPATIONAL EXPOSURES TO HIV AND RECOMMENDATIONS FOR POSTEXPOSURE PROPHYLAXIS

HIV infection can spread through a percutaneous injury, mucosal contact or contact of nonintact skin with blood, tissue, or other body fluids from an infected source. Nonintact skin means exposed skin that is chapped, abraded, or afflicted with dermatitis. Saliva, sputum, tears, sweat, nasal secretions, urine, feces and vomitus are not considered potentially infectious unless they contain blood.

The risk for HIV infection via percutaneous injury increases with increase in quantity of blood from the source person. Percutaneous injury can transmit HIV via:

1. A sharp object (e.g. a needle) visibly contaminated with the patient's blood.
2. A procedure involving a needle being placed directly in a vein or artery, e.g. IV infusion or transfusion or taking out blood.
3. A deep injury.

RECOMMENDED HIV POSTEXPOSURE PROPHYLAXIS (PEP) FOR PERCUTANEOUS INJURIES

For HIV Positive, Class 1 Source

HIV +ve class 1 includes cases with asymptomatic HIV infection or known low viral load (< 1500 RNA copies/ml).

If injury is less severe (injury inflicted with a solid needle or superficial injury like scratches), basic 2-drug PEP is recommended.

If injury is more severe (e.g. large bore hollow needle, needle used in patient's artery or vein, deep puncture, visible blood on device or contact with a large volume of blood has occurred) basic 3-drug PEP is recommended.

For HIV Positive, Class 2 Source

HIV +ve class 2 means symptomatic HIV infection, AIDS, acute seroconversion, or known high viral load. Basic 3-drug PEP is recommended for healthcare workers exposed to class 2 HIV +ve source, irrespective of the severity of sharps injury.

For Source of Unknown HIV Status

Basic 2-drug PEP should be considered for only those cases where source is associated with HIV risk factors. Otherwise, PEP is not warranted. If PEP is administered and later it is determined that source is HIV –ve, PEP should be discontinued.

If the Source is Unknown

The example of such incidents is needle stick injury from sharps waste containers. In such cases, basic 2-drug PEP is recommended only for such settings where there is likely exposure to HIV infected persons. Otherwise PEP is not warranted.

If the Source is HIV –ve

No PEP is recommended, irrespective of the severity of the injury. If drug resistance is a concern, obtain expert consultation. Initiation of PEP should not be delayed pending expert consultation. Because expert consultation alone cannot substitute for face-to-face counseling, resources should be available to provide immediate evaluation and follow-up care for all exposures.

HIV PEP (TABLE 13.7)

If HIV status of the source is unknown, it is recommended to get the source patient immediately tested for HIV. PEP should be administered to the exposed person as soon as possible, preferably within hours of exposure and should be continued for 4 weeks. Because toxic potential of the antiretroviral drugs used in PEP is very high, experts in the field of antiretroviral therapy and transmission of HIV should be consulted before administering PEP. As soon as HIV status of the source patient becomes available,

Table 13.7: Recommended doses of HIV postexposure prophylaxis (PEP) for mucous membrane exposures and nonintact skin exposures

Type of exposure	*Infection status of source*				
	HIV positive, class 1	*HIV positive, class 2*	*Source of unknown HIV status*	*Unknown source*	*HIV negative*
Small volume	Consider basic 2-drug PEP.	Recommend basic 2-drug PEP.	Generally, no PEP warranted.	Generally, no PEP warranted.	No PEP warranted.
Large volume	Recommend basic 2-drug PEP.	Recommend expanded >3-drug PEP.	Generally, no PEP warranted; however, consider basic 2-drug PEP for source with HIV risk factors.	Generally, no PEP warranted; however, consider basic 2-drug PEP in settings in which exposure to HIV-infected persons is likely.	No PEP warranted.

Source: Updated US public health service guidelines for the management of occupational exposures to HIV and recommendations for postexposure prophylaxis, 2005.

it is recommended to reevaluate exposed healthcare worker, as related to decision regarding continuation of PEP.

Selection of Drugs for HIV PEP

Combination regimens using three or more antiretroviral agents have certain advantages over monotherapy and dual-therapy regimens, as proved in HIV infected patients. These are:

a. Combination therapy is more effective in reducing HIV viral load
b. Reduced incidence of opportunistic infections and death, and
c. Delayed onset of drug resistance.

The majority of HIV exposures can be managed by a two-drug combination therapy as the total body viral load is very low as compared to HIV infected source patient. It also improves compliance and chances of completion of full-course of regimen. The recommended two-drug combination regime options are:

1. Two NRTIs (Nucleoside Reverse Transcriptase Inhibitors), e.g. Zidovudine (Retrovir®, AZT, ZDV) + Lamivudine (Epivir®, 3TC) or Emtricitabine (Emtriva, FTC) Stavudine (Zerit™, d4T) + Lamivudine or Emtricitabine.
2. One NRTI and one NtRTI (Nucleotide Analog Reverse Transcriptase Inhibitors), e.g. Tenofovir (Viread®, TDF) + Lamivudine or Emtricitabine.

***Note*:** NRTIs and NtRTIs have the potential to cause lactic acidosis with hepatic steatosis. Also, individual agents have their own toxic effects on various organ systems of body.

Because all antiretroviral agents have been associated with side effects, the toxicity profile of these agents including the frequency, severity, duration and reversibility of side effects, is an important consideration in selection of an HIV PEP regimen.

Follow-up of Exposed Healthcare Personnel

The exposed healthcare worker should receive follow-up counseling, postexposure testing, and medical evaluation in addition to PEP. Postexposure testing is done by EIA for HIV-antibody for more than 6 months after exposure. This is done to observe if seroconversion occurs or not. Follow-up testing should be performed at 6 weeks, 12 weeks and 6 months after exposure. However healthcare workers infected with HCV, after exposure to a source coinfected with HCV and HIV should be monitored for extended period.

Note: Any exposed person, who has developed an illness with symptoms similar to an acute retroviral syndrome, should undergo HIV testing, regardless of the interval since exposure.

Adverse Effects of the Initial PEP Regimen

PEP produces nausea and diarrhea very commonly as adverse effects which can be managed palliatively with the help of anti-emetic and antidiarrheal drugs respectively. For other adverse effects, management can be done by modifying dose interval in terms of either reduction in dose, but more frequent intake per day, or by administering the drug after meals.[92]

OCCUPATIONAL TRANSMISSION OF HCV

Postexposure Management for HCV

A short course of interferon administered during acute hepatitis C is more effective than that during established chronic hepatitis. Moreover, if treatment is administered within 6 months of onset of infection in a case of chronic hepatitis C, it resolves the infection at the same rate as it does during acute hepatitis C.

Management of Exposures to HCV

Anti-HCV level testing should be performed for the sources. If the source is HCV positive, the exposed healthcare worker should undergo the test for baseline level of anti-HCV and ALT activity;

i. Healthcare worker should be followed-up by testing after 4 to 6 months postexposure for anti-HCV and ALT activity.
ii. Testing for HCV- RNA may be performed at 4 to 6 weeks if earlier diagnosis of HCV infection is desired.
    - Confirmatory test for positive results is enzyme immunoassay using supplemental anti-HCV testing (e.g. Recombinant Immunoblot Assay [RIBA]).

The exposed person should be educated about the risk for HCV infection and appropriate counseling, testing, and medical follow-up. For persons exposed to HCV positive blood, IG and antiviral agents are not recommended.[93]

RABIES

People in high risk group, e.g. animal handlers/caretakers, veterinarians or laboratory workers who may be exposed to the rabies virus, should be offered pre-exposure vaccination.

- In addition, pregnant women workers who are exposed to rabies may also be vaccinated.

The rabies vaccine is available as:

Human Diploid Cell Vaccine (HDCV)

Purified Chick Embryo Cell Culture Vaccine (PCECV).

Dose Schedule

A series of three injections is recommended for pre-exposure rabies vaccines administration.

The recommended schedule is 0, 7, 21/28 days.

Dosage: 1 ml injection, in deltoid region.

Individuals, who continue to be at increased risk of contacting rabies, should get booster doses of vaccine every two years to maintain protective antibody levels. Laboratory workers who come in contact with live rabies virus should be tested every six months for adequate antibody levels, and receive boosters as necessary.

Postexposure Rabies Vaccines

The previous immunization status of the individual determines the number of doses required.

Previously unvaccinated people: They should be administered Human Rabies Immunoglobulin (HRIG) along with first dose of 1 ml rabies vaccine as early as possible. HRIG confers protection which persist until rabies vaccine starts working. The dosing schedule is 0, 3, 7, 14 days. For persons with immunosuppression, an additional dose is needed which is administered on 28th day.

Previously vaccinated people: An immunized person is anyone who has received a complete series of vaccine, or a person who has received a pre-exposure or postexposure series of any rabies vaccine who has an adequate rabies antibody level. An immunized person does not require HRIG, only rabies vaccine (HDCV or PCECV) administration is required. It is administered in 2 doses:

1st—Immediately after exposure—1 ml in deltoid region.

2nd—3 days after first dose—1 ml in deltoid region.[18,41]

H1N1 FLU (SWINE FLU)

2009 H1N1, also called as 'swine flu', is a new influenza virus which spreads from person-to-person through coughing, sneezing or talking by people with influenza, by touching a surface or object contaminated with flu viruses. 2009 H1N1 flu was declared a pandemic by WHO.[13]

All healthcare personnel should either wash their hands or use an alcohol based hand rub before and after administering the vaccine.[14]

The H1N1 vaccine protects only against the new H1N1 influenza virus and does not protect against other strains of seasonal flu. Two types of H1N1 vaccines are nasal spray and injectable vaccine. The injectable H1N1 vaccine does not contain an actual live virus; it contains viral proteins. The nasal spray vaccine is a Live Attenuated Virus (LAV) vaccine.[50]

Live Attenuated Intranasal H1N1 Vaccine (Tables 13.8 and 13.9)

Indication

1. Healthy people 2 to 49 years old who are not pregnant.

Contraindications:

1. Allergy to: Previous influenza vaccine
   Eggs, egg protein, gentamicin, gelatin or arginine or other substances in the vaccine
2. Age less than 2 or ≥ 50 years
3. Pregnant ladies
4. Immunocompromised persons

Table 13.8: Recommended doses of vaccine: Time between seasonal and H1N1 doses

	Seasonal nasal (LAIV)	*Seasonal flu shot*
H1N1 Nasal (LAIV)	Minimum two weeks between vaccinations.	May be given in same visit.
H1N1 flu shot	May be given in same visit.	May be given in same visit.

Source: *http://www.sccvote.org/SCC/docs/Public%20Health %20Department%20(DEP)/attachments/FAQ_H1N1_Nasal_Spray_FAQs.pdf*

5. History of Guillain-Barré syndrome (Guillain-Barré syndrome is a rare neurological illness)
6. Long-term medical illness
7. Children or adolescents receiving aspirin therapy.[16,36]

Examples of Intranasal (Nasal Spray) Vaccines

Med-Immune LLC

1. Refrigerated influenza A (H1N1) 2009 monovalent vaccine live is supplied in prefilled unit dose nasal sprayers.
2. Vaccine is stored at 2 to 8°C.
3. Vaccine can be administered along with any other vaccine, but cannot be given with another intranasal vaccine.
4. 0.2 ml dose is contained in the syringe. (0.1 ml per nostril)
5. Dosing is same regardless of age.
6. For children of age group 2 to 9 years, 2 doses are given 3 to 4 weeks apart.
7. For persons aged between 10 to 49 years, 1 dose is sufficient.[90]

Procedure of Administration

1. Make the patient sit in upright position.
2. Remove the rubber tip protector and insert tip just inside nostril.
3. Depress the plunger rapidly until dose divider clip stops.
4. Remove the tip from nose, remove dose divider clip, and administer the remainder dose in opposite nostril.
5. If patient sneezes after vaccine administration, no need to repeat the dose.[49]

Table 13.9: Recommended doses of vaccine: Flu shot or nasal spray?

Age and conditions	*One dose each of seasonal and H1N1 flu vaccines*	*Two doses each of seasonal and H1N1 flu vaccines*	*Ok to get nasal spray?*
0–6 months	No	No	No
6 months–9 years	One dose of seasonal flu vaccine if the child has had seasonal flu vaccination in the past. Two doses of H1N1 flu vaccine are needed.	Two doses of seasonal flu vaccine are needed if this is the first time the child is receiving flu vaccination. Two doses of H1N1 flu vaccine are needed.	No for children younger than two years. Yes, for children older than two years, unless the child has certain conditions. Check below for conditions information.
10–49 years	Yes	No	Can receive nasal spray if healthy and no underlying health conditions.
50 years and older	Flu shot only	No	No
Pregnant women	Flu shot only	No	No
Arthritis	Flu shot only	No	No
Asthma	Flu shot only	Two doses of only flu shot if 6 months–9 years (if first time flu vaccination)	No
HIV/AIDS	Flu shot only	Two doses of only flu shot if 6 months–9 years (if first time flu vaccination)	No
5 years and younger, with a history of	Flu shot only	Two doses of only flu shot if 6 months–5 years (if first time flu vaccination)	No
0–6 months	Recurrent wheezing		

Contd...

Contd...

Age and conditions	*One dose each of seasonal and H1N1 flu vaccines*	*Two doses each of seasonal and H1N1 flu vaccines*	*Ok to get nasal spray?*
Children or adolescents receiving aspirin therapy.	Flu shot only	Two doses of only Flu shot if 6 months to 9 years (if first time flu vaccination)	No
People who have had Guillain-Barré syndrome (GBS) within 6 weeks of getting a flu vaccine.	No	No	No
People who have a severe allergy to chicken eggs or who are allergic to any of the nasal spray vaccine components.	No	No	No

Source: *http://www.flu.gov/individualfamily/vaccination/index.html*

Possible reactions after vaccination are:

- Running or congested nose
- Fever, chills, malaise, myalgia
- Headache, sore throat, nausea, vomiting.[16]

Injection vaccine

Inactivated vaccine or killed virus vaccine is injected into the muscle.

Swine Flu Vaccine Dosage

1. Sanofi Pasteur
   - For infants of 6 to 35 months: Two 0.25 ml doses with one month interval in between.
   - For children 36 months to 9 years: Two 0.5 ml doses with one month interval in between.
   - For children of age ≥ 10 years and adults: A single 0.5 ml dose.

H1N1 Vaccine During Pregnancy or Breastfeeding

The US Centers for Disease Control and Prevention recommend immediate vaccination for all pregnant or breastfeeding mothers. The manufacturers of this vaccine, i.e. Sanofi Pasteur, Inc. does not recommend their vaccine for use in pregnant or lactating women.[86]

Reactions to the Injection Vaccine

a. High fever or behavior changes.
b. Severe allergic reaction in the form of dyspnea, hoarseness or wheezing, pallor, weakness, palpitations or dizziness. The life-threatening allergic reactions occur within few minutes of injection.
c. Mild problems like soreness, redness, tenderness or swelling at injection site, headache, myalgia, nausea, etc. These problems usually begin soon after the injection and last for 1 to 2 days.[12]

Various injection vaccines available

1. **CSL Limited**
   Influenza A (H1N1) 2009 monovalent vaccine contains 15 mcg hemagglutinin per 0.5 ml dose of influenza A/California/7/2009 (H1N1)v-like virus.
2. **Novartis Vaccines and Diagnostics Limited**
   Influenza A (H1N1) 2009 monovalent vaccine is a homogenized, sterile, slightly opalescent suspension in a phosphate buffered saline. Influenza A (H1N1) 2009 monovalent vaccine contains 15 mcg hemagglutinin (HA) per 0.5 ml dose of the following virus strain: A/California/7/2009 (H1N1)v-like virus. The 0.5 ml prefilled syringe presentation does not contain any preservative. However, the 5 ml multidose vial formulation contains thimerosal, a mercury derivative, as a preservative. For each 0.5 ml dose from the multidose vial, 25 mcg mercury is added.
3. **Sanofi Pasteur, Inc.**
   Influenza A (H1N1) 2009 monovalent vaccine contains 15 mcg hemagglutinin (HA) of influenza A/California/07/2009 (H1N1) v-like virus per 0.5 ml dose.[90]

Postexposure antiviral chemoprophylaxis

Pre-exposure prophylaxis in the form of flu vaccine is the first and most important step in preventing flu. Antiviral drugs are a second line of defense against the flu and provide postexposure chemoprophylaxis. When antiviral therapy is indicated, it should be started immediately as waiting for laboratory confirmation of influenza can delay treatment. Also a negative rapid test for influenza does not rule out influenza. The rapid influenza diagnostic tests can be sensitive for 2009 H1N1 virus in the range of 10 to 70 percent.

Postexposure antiviral chemoprophylaxis with either oseltamivir (Tamiflu®) or zanamivir (Relenza®) can be considered for healthcare personnel, public health workers, or first responders who have had a known, unprotected close contact exposure to a source with confirmed, probable, or suspected 2009 H1N1 or seasonal influenza in infective stage. However, to reduce the need for postexposure chemoprophylaxis among healthcare workers, use recommended PPE and other administrative measures (e.g. having ill healthcare personnel stay home, and identification of potentially infectious patients, etc.). Healthcare personnel, who have occupational exposures, should be counseled about the early signs and symptoms of influenza, and advised to immediately contact their healthcare provider for evaluation and possible early treatment if clinical signs or symptoms develop.

Duration of postexposure antiviral chemoprophylaxis is 10 days after the last known exposure.[15] Tamiflu® is available in the form of a tablet or liquid and Relenza® is available as a powder for inhalation.

For treatment of 2009 H1N1 flu, Tamiflu® and Relenza® are usually administered for 5 days. However people hospitalized with flu require treatment for more than 5 days. Flu antiviral drugs work best if started within 2 days of getting sick. However, antiviral drugs can be useful even after two days if:

- The sick person has a greater risk of serious flu complications
- The person has certain symptoms like shortness of breath, chest pain/pressure, dizziness, or confusion
- The person is hospitalized because of the flu.

Most healthy people infected with flu do not need to be treated with antiviral drugs. However, antiviral drugs should be used early to treat flu in very sick people or have a greater chance of getting serious flu complications.[11]

People at greater risk of serious flu complications can include:

- Children, particularly younger than 2 years old.
- Adults aged ≥ 65 years.
- Pregnant women and women up to 2 weeks from parturition.
- People with certain chronic medical conditions (such as heart failure, asthma, chronic lung disease) and immunocompromised people (such as diabetics, HIV infected people).
- People aged less than 19 years receiving long-term aspirin therapy.[15]

Antiviral medicine does not cause harm to a pregnant woman or her unborn baby. Instead, antiviral medicine can help prevent complications such as severe illness and even death. Till now, Tamiflu® is the best medicine to treat pregnant women having 2009 H1N1 flu.

Side Effects of Antiviral Drugs

Tamiflu®—nausea or vomiting (usually occur in the first 2 days of treatment). To reduce these side effects, Tamiflu® can be taken with food.

Relenza®—dizziness, sinusitis, runny or stuffy nose, cough, diarrhea, nausea, or headache, wheezing and difficulty in breathing in people with lung disease.

Tamiflu® or Relenza® can rarely cause confusion and abnormal behavior in people with the flu, mostly children. It is advised to closely monitor persons taking these drugs for signs of unusual behavior or problems thinking clearly. And report this behavior immediately to a healthcare provider.[11]

CHAPTER 14 Infection Control Practices in Waste Management

INFECTION CONTROL

Infection control refers to policies and procedures used to minimize the risk of spreading infections, specially in hospitals and human or animal healthcare facilities.

Why do we Need Infection Control?

We need infection control to:

- Reduce the occurrence of infectious diseases. These diseases (usually bacterial or viral) can be spread by human to human contact, animal to human contact, human contact with an infected surface, airborne transmission, and as food or water.
- Reduce the hospital acquired infections, also called as nosocomial infections. The prevalence of such infections is approximately 5 percent among all hospital patients.[34]

It is very important to note and recognize that infection control is the responsibility of all healthcare professionals—doctors, nurses, therapists, pharmacists, engineers and others. Preventing nosocomial infections requires a hygienic and sanitized environment and maintenance of good practices and use of protective gear.

Routine cleaning of the health facility is absolutely essential, as that will keep the environment free from dust and soil. Running water, soaps or antiseptic and facilities for drying without contamination, are required for healthcare workers to maintain cleanliness at all times. As a general practice of maintaining good hygiene, the floors of the healthcare facility should be first swabbed with a wet cloth, then swept to remove grits to avoid dust carrying pathogens from rising into the air and, finally, swabbed with a disinfectant solution. The swab cloth should be washed with detergent after every use. Infected linen in the hospital should be carefully packed in plastic bags, taken to the washing area, stored in bleach solution and then washed with the usual cleaning agents.[55]

Who Should Use Personal Protective Equipment?

All the persons entering the isolation room/area should use personal protective equipment. These include:

- Healthcare workers, providing direct patient care (e.g. doctors, nurses, radiographers, physiotherapists)
- All support staff including medical assistants and cleaning staff
- Attendants, family members or visitors
- All laboratory workers, as they handle specimens from the patients
- All workers engaged in sterilization of equipment that requires decontamination.

Infection control practices can be grouped in two categorized as:

1. *Standard precautions*: These are basic infection control precautions, which must be applied to each and every patient at all times, regardless of his diagnosis or infectious status.
2. *Additional (transmission-based) precautions*: These are infection control precautions specific to modes of transmission (airborne, droplet and contact) and are applied in addition to standard precautions, wherever necessary.

STANDARD PRECAUTIONS

During treatment of every patient in a healthcare facility, application of the same "standard" precautions requires work practices essential to provide a high level of protection to patients, healthcare workers and visitors.

These standard precautions include the following:

1. Hand hygiene, i.e. handwashing and antisepsis.
2. Use of appropriate personal protective equipment while handling organs/body tissue, blood, body substances and excretions and secretions.

3. Appropriate safe and careful handling of patient care equipment and soiled linen.
4. Prevention of needle stick/sharp injuries.
5. Environmental cleaning and spills-management.
6. Scientific handling of waste.

Handwashing and Antisepsis (Hand Hygiene)

Microorganisms are acquired on the hands during daily duties, contact with blood, body fluids, secretions, excretions and known/ unknown contaminated surfaces or equipment. Appropriate hand hygiene can minimize these vectors of diseases.

It is recommended to wash or decontaminate hands:

- After contact with any blood/body fluids/excretions/secretions and contaminated surfaces or equipment.
- Between various tasks and procedures on the same patient so as to prevent cross contamination between different sites of body.
- Between contact with different patients.
- Immediately after removing gloves using a plain soap antimicrobial agent or waterless antiseptic agent.

Use of Personal Protective Equipment (Fig. 14.1)

Personal protective equipment provides a physical barrier between external microorganisms and the wearer. It renders protection by preventing microorganisms from contaminating clothing, hands, eyes, hair and shoes, and by preventing transmission of these microorganisms to other patients and staff.

Full Personal Protective Equipment

- Hair cover (cap)
- Eyewears (goggles)
- Face mask
- Gloves
- Gown
- Apron
- Shoe covers.

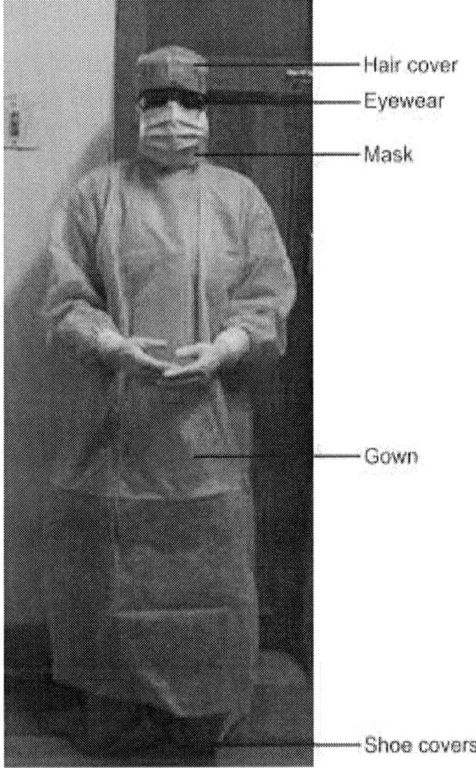

Fig. 14.1: Full personal protective equipment

Personal protective equipment should be used by:

Healthcare workers who provide direct care to patients (e.g. doctors, nurse, etc.) and those who work in conditions where there are chances of contact with blood, body fluids, excretions or secretions, e.g.

- Support staff including medical aides, cleaners, and laundry staff can have contact with blood, body fluids, secretions and excretions
- Laboratory staff
- Family members and attendants who provide care to patients and contact blood, body fluids, secretions and excretions.

Principles for Use of Personal Protective Equipment

Although personal protective equipment reduces the risk of acquiring an infection, it does not eliminate the risk completely. It must be used in an effective and correct manner and every time when there are chances of contact with blood and body fluids of all patients. Continuous availability of personal protective equipment and adequate training for its proper use are essential requirements. Standard procedure for cleaning and disinfection of reusable equipments used for personal protective equipment are given in Table 14.1.

The following principles guide the use of personal protective equipment:

a. The basis for selection of personal protective equipment should be the risk of exposure. Healthcare workers should make an assessment if they are at risk of exposure to blood, body fluids excretions or secretions and select the items of personal protective equipment accordingly.
b. Contaminated (used) personal protective equipment should not contact any surfaces, clothing or people outside the patient care area.
c. Discard used personal protective equipment in appropriate disposal bags, as per protocol of the healthcare establishment.
d. Do not share personal protective equipment.
e. Personal protective equipment should be completely changed.
f. Thoroughly wash hands each time you leave a patient to attend to another patient or another duty.

Gloves (Fig. 14.2)

- Wear clean and nonsterile gloves while touching blood, body fluids, mucous membranes, secretions or excretions
- Change gloves between contacts with different patients to prevent cross contamination between patients
- Also, change gloves between tasks/procedures on the same patient so that cross contamination between different body sites is prevented.

Table 14.1: Standard procedure for cleaning and disinfection of reusable equipments used for personal protective equipment

Equipment	*Standard procedure*	*Comments*
Apron Use of disposable apron is recommended.	If reusable: Clean with detergent and water, dry, disinfect with 70% alcohol.	If disposable: Discard in appropriate waste bag according to the healthcare facility guidelines.
N 95 or standard surgical mask. Use disposable mask only.		Discard in appropriate waste bag according to the healthcare facility guidelines.
HEPA (PIOO) mask. Use disposable filters only.	Separate the filters from the mask and discard the filter. Clean the mask with detergent and water dry and disinfect with 70% alcohol before reuse.	Discard the filters in appropriate bag according to the healthcare facility guidelines.
Eye Protector/goggles/face shield. Use of disposable goggles is recommended.	If reusable: Clean with detergent and water, dry, and disinfect with 70% alcohol or soak in 1% hypochlorite solution for 20 minutes and rinse and dry.	If disposable: Discard in appropriate waste bag according to the healthcare facility guidelines.
Gown Use of disposable gown is recommended.	If reusable: Launder as per the healthcare facility guidelines for soiled linen. For example: Launder in hot water (70 to 80°C) if possible. **OR** Soak in clean water with bleaching powder 0.5% for 30 minutes. Wash again with detergent and water to remove the bleach.	If disposable: Discard in appropriate waste bag according to the healthcare facility guidelines. If reusable: Ideally dry in a clothesdrier or in the sun.

Contd...

Contd...

Equipment	*Standard procedure*	*Comments*
Cap Use of disposable cap is recommended.	If reusable: Launder as per the healthcare facility guidelines for soiled linen. For example: Launder in hot water (70 to 80°C) if possible. **OR** Soak in clean water with bleaching powder 0.5% for 30 minutes. Wash again with detergent and water to remove the bleach.	If disposable: Discard in appropriate waste bag.Seal the bag. If reusable: Ideally dry in a clothes drier or in the sun
Gloves Use disposable gloves only.		Discard in the appropriate waste bag according to the healthcare facility guidelines.

Source: *Practical Guidelines for infection control in healthcare facilities (WHO)*

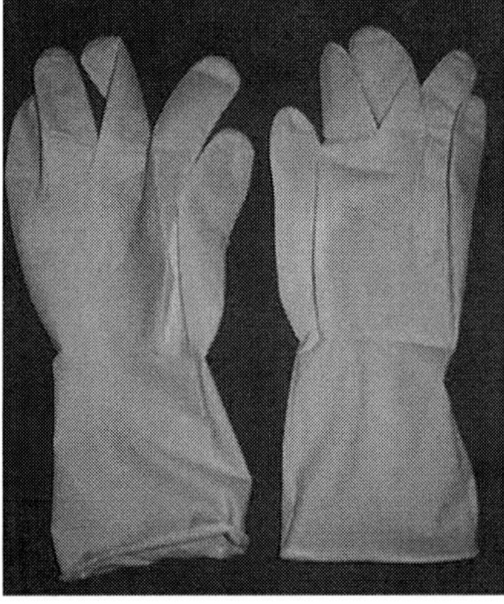

Fig. 14.2: Gloves

- Remove gloves immediately after use and before attending to another patient
- Wash hands immediately after removing gloves using a plain soap, antimicrobial agent or waterless antiseptic agent
- Disposable gloves should not be reused. Instead, they should be disposed of according to the healthcare facility protocol.

Note: It is important to use personal protective equipment effectively, correctly and at all times where contact with patient's blood, body fluids, excretions and secretions may occur.

Masks

- A face mask should be worn to protect mucous membranes of the mouth and nose when during procedures that are likely to generate splashes of blood, body fluids, secretions or excretions
- Surgical masks should be preferred over cotton, material or gauze masks because surgical masks have been designed to resist fluids to varying degrees depending on the design of the material in the mask
- Never reuse disposable masks. Instead, they should be disposed of according to the protocol of healthcare facility.

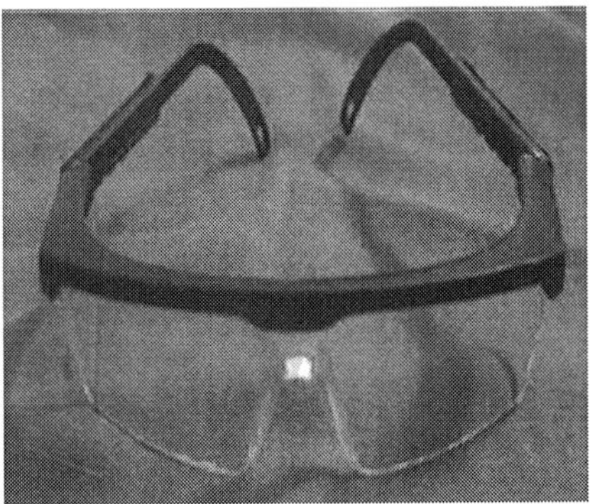

Fig. 14.3: Protective eyewear

Protective Eyewear/Goggles/Visors/Face Shield (Fig. 14.3)

The mucous membranes of the eyes need to be protected when conducting procedures that are likely to generate splashes of blood, body fluids, secretions or excretions. For protection of eyes, wear protective eyewear/goggles/visors/face shields. If disposable, discard appropriately.

Gowns and Plastic Aprons

- Wear a clean, nonsterile gown to protect the skin and prevent soiling of clothing during procedures that are likely to generate splashes of blood and other body fluids, secretions or excretions
- Impermeable gowns are preferable
- A plastic apron worn on top of the gown renders protection against exposure to blood, body fluids, secretions and excretions
- Remove a soiled or wet gown as soon as possible
- Reusable gowns and aprons appropriately laundered, according to the hospital guidelines
- Never reuse disposable gowns and aprons. Instead, they should be disposed of according to the healthcare facility's protocol.

Caps and Boots/Shoe Covers

- Disposable caps and boots are required where there are chances of splashing, spillage or leakage of the patient's blood, body fluids, secretions or excretions, onto the hair or shoes of the healthcare worker.

- Do not reuse disposable caps. They should be discarded according to the healthcare facility protocol
- Decontaminate reusable boots
- Discard boots/shoe covers after use according to the healthcare facility protocol.

Handling of Patient Care Equipment and Soiled Linen

Patient Care Equipment

Handle patient care equipment soiled with blood, body fluids secretions or excretions with care in order to prevent exposure to skin and mucous membranes, clothing and the environment.

Ensure all reusable equipment is cleaned and reprocessed appropriately before being used on another patient.

Linen

Handle, transport and process used linen that is soiled with blood, body fluids, secretions or excretions with care to ensure that there is no leaking of fluid.

Prevention of Needle Stick/Sharps Injuries

- Be careful when using needles, scalpels and other sharp instruments or equipment, and when cleaning sharp reusable instruments or equipment
- Never recap or bend needles
- Place used disposable syringes and needles, scalpel blades and other sharp items in a puncture-resistant container
- The sharps container should be placed close to the site of their use and generation
- The container must have a lid that closes.

Note: Sharps must be appropriately decontaminated and/or destroyed according to the national standards or guidelines.

ADDITIONAL (TRANSMISSION-BASED) PRECAUTIONS

Additional (transmission-based) precautions are taken in addition to standard precautions. Additional, i.e.

- Airborne precautions
- Droplet precautions
- Contact precautions.

Airborne Precautions

Design of airborne precautions is such that they reduce the transmission of diseases spread by the airborne route. Airborne transmission occurs when droplet nuclei or evaporated droplets measuring <5 micron in size are disseminated in the air that can remain suspended in the air for long periods time. Droplet nuclei (the residuals of droplets) when suspended in the air, dry and produce particles of 1 to 5 microns that can remain suspended indefinitely in the air. Diseases spread by this mode include open/active pulmonary tuberculosis (TB), pulmonary plague, chickenpox, measles and hemorrhagic fever with pneumonia.

The following precautions need to be taken:

I. Implementation of standard precautions.
II. Placing patient in a single room that has a monitored negative airflow pressure called as a "negative pressure room". The air from this room should be either discharged to the outdoors or specially filtered before circulating it to other areas of healthcare facility.
III. Keeping doors of this room closed always.
IV. All the persons entering the room must wear a special, high filtration, particulate respirator (e.g. N 95) mask (Fig. 14.4).
V. Limiting the movement and transport of the patient from the room for essential purposes only. If transport is necessary, minimize dispersal of droplet nuclei by masking the patient.

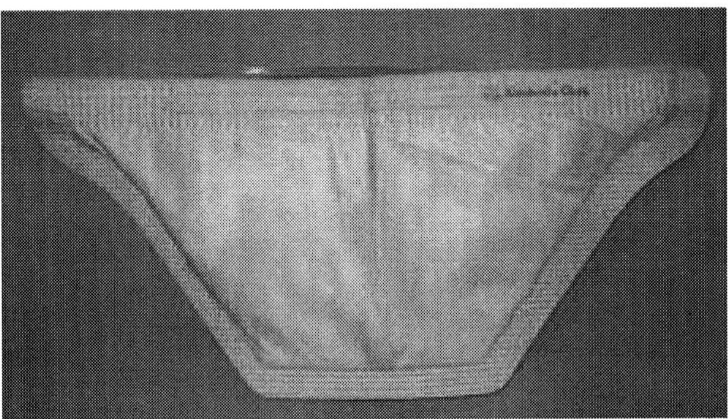

Fig. 14.4: N 95 mask

Droplet Precautions

Diseases transmitted by this route include pneumonias, diphtheria, meningitis, influenza type B, mumps, pertussis, etc. Adequate contact between the mucous membranes of the nose, mouth or conjunctivae of a susceptible person and large particle droplets (> 5 microns) results in droplet transmission. These droplets are usually generated from the infected person during coughing, sneezing and talking. These may also generate when healthcare workers perform procedures such as suction.

Personal Protective Equipment Used for SARS (Severe Acute Respiratory Syndrome)

If used correctly, personal protective equipment reduces the risk of infection. The items included in PPE are:

- Gloves (nonsterile)
- Mask (N95 preferable)
- Protective eyewear/goggles/visors/face shields
- Plastic apron if chances of splashing of blood, body fluids, excretions and secretions are there
- Long sleeved cuffed gown
- Cap (in high-risk situations of increased aerosols).

Contact Precautions

Diseases transmitted by this route include infection or colonization with multiple antibiotic resistant organisms, enteric infections and skin infections.

The following precautions are required to be taken:

- Implementation of standard precautions
- Place patient in a single room (or in a room with another similarly infected patient)
- Always wear clean, nonsterile gloves when entering the room
- Wear a clean, nonsterile gown when entering the room if substantial contact with the patient, surfaces or items in the patient's room is anticipated
- Limit the patient's movement and transport from the room for essential purposes only. If transportation is required, use precautions to minimize the risk of transmission.[98]

Appendix

THE BIOMEDICAL WASTE (MANAGEMENT AND HANDLING) RULES, 1998

MINISTRY OF ENVIRONMENT AND FORESTS NOTIFICATION
New Delhi, 20th July, 1998

[1]**SO 630(E)**—Whereas a notification in exercise of the powers conferred by Sections 6, 8 and 25 of the Environment (Protection) Act, 1986 (29 of 1986) was published in the Gazette vide SO 746(E), dated 16 October, 1997 inviting objections from the public within 60 days from the date of the publication of the said notification on the Biomedical Waste (Management and Handling) Rules, 1998 and whereas all objections received were duly considered.

Now, therefore, in exercise of the powers conferred by Section 6, 8 and 25 of the Environment (Protection) Act, 1986 the Central Government hereby notifies the rules for the management and handling of biomedical waste.

1. SHORT TITLE AND COMMENCEMENT

1. These rules may be called the Biomedical Waste (Management and Handling) Rules, 1998.
2. They shall come into force on the date of their publication in the official Gazette.

2. APPLICATION

These rules apply to all persons who generate, collect, receive, store, transport, treat, dispose, or handle biomedical waste in any form.

3. DEFINITIONS

In these rules unless the context otherwise requires:

1. "**Act**" means the Environment (Protection) Act, 1986 (29 of 1986);
2. "**Animal House**" means a place where animals are reared/kept for experiments or testing purposes;

---

[1]As published in Gazette of India, Extraordinary Part II Section 3, Subsection (ii), vide notification SO 630(E), dated 20.7.1998.

3. **"Authorization"** means permission granted by the prescribed authority for the generation, collection, reception, storage, transportation, treatment, disposal and/or any other form of handling of biomedical waste in accordance with these rules and any guidelines issued by the Central Government.
4. **"Authorized person"** means an occupier or operator authorized by the prescribed authority to generate, collect, receive, store, transport, treat, dispose and/or handle biomedical waste in accordance with these rules and any guidelines issued by the Central Government.
5. **"Biomedical waste"** means any waste, which is generated during the diagnosis, treatment or immunization of human beings or animals or in research activities pertaining thereto or in the production or testing of biologicals, and including categories mentioned in Schedule I.
6. **"Biologicals"** means any preparation made from organisms or microorganisms or product of metabolism and biochemical reactions intended for use in the diagnosis, immunization or the treatment of human beings or animals or in research activities pertaining thereto.
7. **"Biomedical waste treatment facility"** means any facility wherein treatment disposal of biomedical waste or processes incidental to such treatment or disposal is carried out [1][and includes common treatment facilities].

   [2][(7a) **'Form'** means Form appended to these rules;]
8. **"Occupier"** in relation to any institution generating biomedical waste, which includes a hospital, nursing home, clinic dispensary, veterinary institution, animal house, pathological laboratory, blood bank by whatever name called, means a person who has control over mat institution and/or its premises.
9. **"Operator of a biomedical waste facility"** means a person who owns or controls or operates a facility for the collection, reception, storage, transport, treatment, disposal or any other form of handling of biomedical waste.
10. **"Schedule"** means schedule appended to these rules.

---

[1]Added by Rule 2(i) of the Biomedical Waste (M&H) (Second Amendment) Rules, 2000 notified vide notification No. SO 545(E), dated 2.6.2000 and came into force wef 2.6.2000.

[2]Inserted by Rule 2 (ii) of the Biomedical Waste (M&H) (Second Amendment) rules, 2000 notified vide Notification No. SO 545(E), dated 2.6.2000 and came into force wef 2.6.2000.

4. DUTY OF OCCUPIER

It shall be the duty of every occupier of an institution generating biomedical waste which includes a hospital, nursing home, clinic, dispensary, veterinary institution, animal house, pathological laboratory, blood bank by whatever name called to take all steps to ensure mat such waste is handled without any adverse effect to human health and the environment.

5. TREATMENT AND DISPOSAL

1. Biomedical waste shall be treated and disposed off in accordance with Schedule I, and in compliance with the standards prescribed in Schedule V.
2. Every occupier, where required, shall set up in accordance with the time-schedule in Schedule VI, requisite biomedical waste treatment facilities like incinerator, autoclave, microwave system for the treatment of waste, or, ensure requisite treatment of waste at a common waste treatment facility or any other waste treatment facility.

6. SEGREGATION, PACKAGING, TRANSPORTATION AND STORAGE

1. Biomedical waste shall not be mixed with other wastes.
2. Biomedical waste shall be segregated into containers/bags at the point of generation in accordance with Schedule II prior to its storage, transportation, treatment and disposal. The containers shall be labeled according to Schedule III.
3. If a container is transported from the premises where biomedical waste is generated to any waste treatment facility outside the premises, the container shall, apart from the label prescribed in Schedule III, also carry information prescribed in Schedule IV.
4. Notwithstanding anything contained in the Motor Vehicles Act, 1988, or rules thereunder, untreated biomedical waste shall be transported only in such vehicle as may be authorized for the purpose by the competent authority as specified by the Government.
5. No untreated biomedical waste shall be kept stored beyond a period of 48 hours:

   Provided mat if for any reason it becomes necessary to store the waste beyond such period, the authorized person must take permission of the prescribed authority and take measures to ensure that the waste does not adversely affect human health and the environment.

[1]6. The Municipal body of the area shall continue to pick up and transport segregated nonbiomedical solid waste generated in hospitals and nursing homes, as well as duly treated biomedical wastes for disposal at municipal dump site.

7. PRESCRIBED AUTHORITY

[2](1)[3] [Save as otherwise provide, the prescribed authority for enforcement] of the provisions of these rules shall be the State Pollution Control Boards in respect of States and the Pollution Control Committees in respect of the Union Territories and all pending cases with a prescribed authority appointed earlier shall stand transferred to the concerned State Pollution Control Board, or as the case may be, the Pollution Control Committees.

[4](1A) The prescribed authority for enforcement of the provisions of these rules in respect of all healthcare establishments including hospitals, nursing homes, clinics, dispensaries, veterinary institutions, Animal houses, pathological laboratories and blood banks of the Armed Forces under the Ministry of Defence shall be the Director General, Armed Forces Medical Services.

2. The prescribed authority for the State or Union Territory shall be appointed within one month of the coming into force of these rules.
3. The prescribed authority shall function under the supervision and control of the respective Government of the State or Union Territory.
4. The prescribed authority shall on receipt of Form I make such enquiry as it deems fit and if it is satisfied mat the applicant possesses the necessary capacity to handle biomedical waste in accordance with these rules, grant or renew an authorization as the case may be.
5. An authorization shall be granted for a period of three years, including an initial trial period of one year from the date of issue. Thereafter, an application shall be made by the occupier/operator for renewal. All such subsequent authorization shall be for a period of three years. A provisional authorization will be granted for the trial period, to enable the occupier/operator to demonstrate the capacity of the facility.

---

[1]Inserted by Rule 3 of the Biomedical Waste (M&H) (Second Amendment) Rules, 2000 vide notification SO 545(E), dated 2.6.2000.

[2]Substituted by Rule 4 of the Biomedical Waste (M&H) (Second Amendment) Rules, 2000 vide notification SO 545(E), dated 2.6.2000.

[3]Substituted by Rule 2 (a) of the Biomedical Waste (M&H) (Amendment) Rules, 2003 vide notification SO 1069(E), dated 17.9.2003.

[4]Inserted subrule (1A) by Rule 2(b), ibid.

6. The prescribed authority may after giving reasonable opportunity of being heard to the applicant and for reasons thereof to be recorded in writing, refuse to grant or renew authorization.
7. Every application for authorization shall be disposed off by the prescribed authority within ninety days from the date of receipt of the application.
8. The prescribed authority may cancel or suspend an authorization, if for reasons, to be recorded in writing, the occupier/operator has failed to comply with any provision of the Act or these rules:

Provided that no authorization shall be cancelled or suspended without giving a reasonable opportunity to the occupier/operator of being heard.

8. AUTHORIZATION

1. Every occupier of an institution generating, collecting, receiving, storing, transporting, treating, disposing and/or handling biomedical waste in any other manner, except such occupier of clinics, dispensaries, pathological laboratories, blood banks providing treatment/service to less than 1000 (one thousand) patients per month, shall make an application in Form I to the prescribed authority for grant of authorization.
2. Every operator of a biomedical waste facility shall make an application in Form I to the prescribed authority for grant of authorization.
3. Every application in Form I for grant of authorization shall be accompanied by a fee as may be prescribed by the Government of the State or Union Territory.

[1](4) The authorization to operate a facility shall be issued in Form IV, subject to conditions laid therein and such other condition, as the prescribed authority, may consider it necessary.

9. ADVISORY COMMITTEE

[2](1) The Government of every State/Union Territory shall constitute an advisory committee. The Committee will include experts in the field of medical and health, animal husbandry and veterinary

---

[1]Inserted by Rule 5 of the Biomedical Waste (M&H) (Second Amendment) Rules, 2000 vide notification SO 545(E), dated 2.6.2000.

[2]Renumbered as Subrule (1) by Rule 3 of the Biomedical Waste (M&H) (Amendment) Rules, 2003 notified vide Notification No. SO 1069(E), dated 17.9.2003.

sciences, environmental management, municipal administration, and any other related department or organization including non-governmental organizations [1][***]. As and when required, the committee shall advise the Government of the State/Union Territory and the prescribed authority about matters related to the implementation of these rules.

[2](2) Notwithstanding anything contained in subrule (1), the Ministry of Defence shall constitute in that Ministry, an Advisory Committee consisting of the following in respect of all healthcare establishments including hospitals, nursing homes, clinics, dispensaries, veterinary institutions, animal houses, pathological laboratories and blood banks of the Armed Forces under the Ministry of Defence, to advise the Director General, Armed Forces Medical Services and the Ministry of Defence in matters relating to implementation of these rules, namely:

1. Additional Director General of Armed Forces Medical Services .... Chairman
2. A representative of the Ministry of Defence not below the rank of Deputy Secretary, to be nominated by that Ministry .... Member
3. A representative of the Ministry of Environment and Forests not below the rank of Deputy Secretary To be nominated by mat Ministry. .... Member
4. A representative of the Indian Society of Hospitals Waste Management, Pune .... Member

[3][9A. MONITORING OF IMPLEMENTATION OF THE RULES IN ARMED FORCES HEALTHCARE ESTABLISHMENTS

1. The Central Pollution Control Board shall monitor the implementation of these rules in respect of all the Armed Forces healthcare establishments under the Ministry of Defence.
2. After giving prior notice to the Director General Armed Forces Medical Services, the Central Pollution Control Board along with

[1]Omitted by Rule 6 of the Biomedical Waste (M&H) (Second Amendment) Rules, 2000 vide notification SO 545(E), dated 2.6.2000.

[2]Inserted subrule (2) by Rule 3 of the Biomedical Waste (M&H) (Amendment) Rules, 2003 notified vide Notification No. SO 1069(E), dated 17.9.2003.

[3]Inserted Rule 9A by Rule 4 of the Biomedical Waste (M&H) (Amendment) Rules, 2003 notified vide Notification No. SO I069(E), dated 17.9.2003.

one or more representatives of the Advisory Committee constituted under subrule (2) of rule 9 may, if it considers it necessary, inspect any Armed Forces healthcare establishments.

10. ANNUAL REPORT

Every occupier/operator shall submit an annual report to the prescribed authority in Form II by 31 January every year, to include information about the categories and quantities of biomedical wastes handled during the preceding year. The prescribed authority shall send misinformation in a compiled form to the Central Pollution Control Board by 31 March every year.

11. MAINTENANCE OF RECORDS

1. Every authorized person shall maintain records related to the generation, collection, reception, storage, transportation, treatment, disposal and/or any form of handling of biomedical waste in accordance with these rules and any guidelines issued.
2. All records shall be subject to inspection and verification by the prescribed authority at any time.

12. ACCIDENT REPORTING

When any accident occurs at any institution or facility or any other site where biomedical waste is handled or during transportation of such waste, the authorized person shall report the accident in Form III to the prescribed authority forthwith.

13. APPEAL

[1](1)[2] [Save as otherwise provided in subrule (2), any person] aggrieved by an order made by the prescribed authority under these rules may, within thirty days from the date on which the order is communicated to him, prefer an appeal [3][in form V] to such authority as the Government of State/Union Territory may mink fit to constitute:

---

[1]Renumbered as subrule (1) by Rule 5 (a) of the Biomedical Wastes (M&H) (Amendment) Rules, 2003 notified vide Notification No. SO 1069(E), dated 17.9.2003.

[2]Substituted by Rule 5(a), ibid.

[3]Inserted by Rule 7 of the Biomedical Waste (M&H) (Second Amendment) Rules, 2000 vide notification SO 545 (E), dated 2.6.2000.

Provided that the authority may entertain the appeal after the expiry of the said period of thirty days if it is satisfied that the appellant was prevented by sufficient cause from filing the appeal in time.

[1](2) Any person aggrieved by an order of the Director General, Armed Forces Medical Services under these rules may, within thirty days from the date on which the order is communicated to him prefer an appeal to the Central Government in the Ministry of Environment and Forests.

[2]14. COMMON DISPOSAL/INCINERATION SITES

Without prejudice to rule 5 of these rules, the Municipal Corporations, Municipal Boards or Urban Local Bodies, as the case may be, shall be responsible for providing suitable common disposal/incineration sites. for the biomedical wastes generated in the area under their jurisdiction and in areas outside the jurisdiction of any municipal body, it shall be the responsibility of the occupier generating biomedical waste/operator of a biomedical waste treatment facility to arrange for suitable sites individually or in association, so as to comply with the provisions of these rules.

[1]Inserted subrule (2) by Rule 5(b) of the Biomedical Waste (M&H) (Amendment) Rules, 2003 notified vide Notification No. SO I069(E), dated 17.9.2003.

[2]Inserted by Rule 8 of the Biomedical Waste (M&H) (Second Amendment) Rules, 2000 notified vide SO 545(E), dated 2.6.2000.

SCHEDULE I
(See Rule 5)
CATEGORIES OF BIOMEDICAL WASTE

[1][Waste category No.]	Waste category [2][type]	Treatment and disposal [3][option +]
Category No.1	**Human anatomical waste** (human tissues, organs, body parts)	Incineration@/deep burial*
Category No. 2	**Animal waste** (animal tissues, organs, body parts carcasses, bleeding parts, fluid, blood and experimental animals used in research, waste generated by veterinary hospitals, colleges discharge from hospitals, animal houses).	Incineration@/deep burial*
Category No. 3	**Microbiology and biotechnology wastes** (Wastes from laboratory cultures, stocks or specimens of microorganisms live or attenuated vaccines, human and animal cell culture used in research and infectious agents from research and industrial laboratories, wastes from production of biologicals, toxins, dishes and devices used for transfer of cultures).	Local autoclaving/ microwaving/incineration@
Category No. 4	**Waste sharps** (Needles, syringes, scalpels, blades, glass, etc. that may cause puncture and cuts. This includes both used and unused sharps).	Disinfection (chemical treatment@@/autoclaving /microwaving and mutilation /shredding ##
Category No. 5	**Discarded medicines and cytotoxic drugs** (Wastes comprising of outdated, contaminated and discarded medicines)	Incineration@/destruction and drugs disposal in secured landfills.

Contd...

[1]Substituted by Rule 9(i) of the Biomedical Waste (M&H) (Second Amendment) Rules, 2000 notified vide SO 545(E), dated 2.6.2000.

[2]Added by Rule 9(ii), ibid.

[3]Substituted by Rule 9 (iii), ibid.

Contd...

[1][*Waste category No.]*	*Waste category* [2][*type]*	*Treatment and disposal* [3][*option +]*
Category No. 6	**[1][Soiled] waste** (Items contaminated with blood, and body fluids including cotton, dressings, soiled plaster casts, lines beddings, other material contaminated with blood).	Incineration @ autoclaving/ microwaving.
Category No. 7	**Solid waste** (Wastes generated from disposable items other than the waste [2][sharps] such as tubings, catheters, intravenous sets, etc.)	Disinfection by chemical treatment@@ autoclaving/ microwaving and mutilation/shredding##.
Category No. 8	**Liquid waste** (Waste generated from laboratory and washing, cleaning, house-keeping and disinfecting activities).	Disinfection by chemical treatment @@ and discharge into drains.
Category No. 9	**Incineration ash** (Ash from incineration of any biomedical waste).	Disposal in municipal landfill.
Category No. 10	**Chemical waste** (Chemicals used in production of biologicals, chemicals used in disinfection, as insecticides, etc.)	Chemical treatment @@ and discharge into drains for liquids and secured landfill for solids.

@@ Chemicals treatment using at least 1% hypochlorite solution or any other equivalent chemical reagent. It must be ensured that chemical treatment ensures disinfection.

Mutilation/shredding must be such so as to prevent unauthorized reuse.

@ There will be no chemical pretreatment before incineration. Chlorinated plastics shall not be incinerated.

* Deep burial shall be an option available only in towns with population less than five lakhs and in rural areas.

[3][+ Options given above are based on available technologies. Occupier/ operator wishing to use other State-of-the-art technologies shall approach the Central Pollution Control Board to get the standards laid down to enable the prescribed authority to consider grant of authorization].

[1]Substituted by rule 9(iv), ibid.

[2]Substituted by Rule 9 (v) of the Biomedical Waste (M&H) (Second Amendment) Rules, 2000 notified vide SO 545(E), dated 2.6.2000.

[3]Substituted by Rule 9 (iii) of the Biomedical Waste (M&H) (Second Amendment) Rules, 2000 notified vide SO 545 (E), dated 2.6.2000.

SCHEDULE II

(See Rule 6)

COLOR CODING AND TYPE OF CONTAINER FOR DISPOSAL OF BIOMEDICAL WASTES

Color coding	*Type of container*	*Waste category*	*Treatment options as per schedule I*
Yellow	Plastic bag	Cat.1, Cat. 2, Cat. 3, Cat. 6	Incineration/deep burial
Red	Disinfected container/plastic bag	Cat. 3, Cat. 6, Cat. 7	Autoclaving/microwaving/ chemical treatment
Blue/white translucent	Plastic bag/puncture proof container	Cat. 4, Cat. 7	Autoclaving/microwaving/ chemical treatment and destruction/shredding
Black	Plastic bag	Cat. 5, Cat. 9 and Cat. 10 (Solid)	Disposal in secured landfill

Notes:

1. Color coding of waste categories with multiple treatment options as defined in Schedule I, shall be selected depending on treatment option chosen, which shall be as specified in Schedule I.
2. Waste collection bags for waste types needing incineration shall not be made of chlorinated plastics.
3. Categories 8 and 10 (liquid) do not require containers/bags.
4. Category 3 if disinfected locally need not be put in containers/bags.

SCHEDULE III
(See Rule 6)

LABEL FOR BIOMEDICAL WASTE CONTAINERS/BAGS

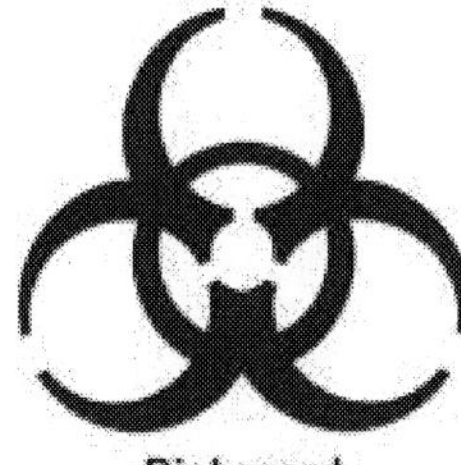

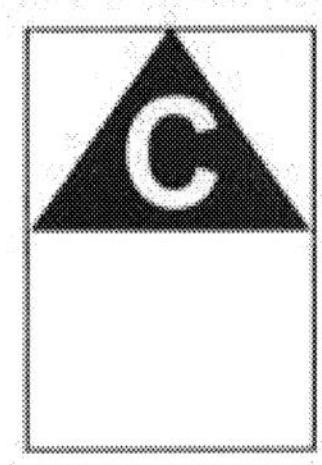

Handle With Care

Note: Label shall be nonwashable and prominently visible.

SCHEDULE IV

(See Rule 6)

LABEL FOR TRANSPORT OF BIOMEDICAL WASTE CONTAINERS/BAGS

Day........... Month...................

Year.......................................

Date of generation...................

Waste category No..........................

Waste class

Waste description

Sender's Name and Address	**Receiver's Name and Address**
Phone No.	Phone No. ....
Telex No.	Telex No. ....
Fax No.	Fax No. ....
Contact person................	Contact person.......................

In case of emergency please contact:

Name and address

Phone No.

Note: Label shall be nonwashable and prominently visible.

SCHEDULE V
(See Rule 5 and Schedule I)
STANDARDS FOR TREATMENT AND DISPOSAL OF BIOMEDICAL WASTES

STANDARDS FOR INCINERATORS

All incinerators shall meet the following operating and emission standards:

A. Operating Standards

1. Combustion efficiency (CE) shall be at least 99.00 percent.
2. The Combustion efficiency is computed as follows:

$$CE = \frac{\% \, CO_2}{\% \, CO_2 + \% \, CO} \times 100$$

3. The temperature of the primary chamber shall be 800 ± 50°C.
4. The secondary chamber gas residence time shall be at least 1 second at 1050 ± 50°C, with minimum 3 percent oxygen in the stack gas.

B. Emission Standards

	Parameters	Concentration mg/Nm^3 at (12% CO_2 correction)
1.	Particulate matter	150
2.	Nitrogen oxides	450
3.	HCl	50

4. Minimum stack height shall be 30 meters above ground.
5. Volatile organic compounds in ash shall not be more man 0.01 percent.

Note:

- Suitably designed pollution control devices should be installed/retrofitted with the incinerator to achieve the above emission limits, if necessary.
- Wastes to be incinerated shall not be chemically treated with any chlorinated disinfectants.
- Chlorinated plastics shall not be incinerated.
- Toxic metals in incineration ash shall be limited within the regulatory quantities as defined under the Hazardous Waste (Management and Handling) Rules, 1989.
- Only low sulfur fuel like LDO/LSHS/Diesel shall be used as fuel in the incinerator.

STANDARDS FOR WASTE AUTOCLAVING

The autoclave should be dedicated for the purposes of disinfecting and treating biomedical waste.

I. When operating a gravity flow autoclave, medical waste shall be subjected to:
   i. A temperature of not less man 121°C and pressure of 15 pounds per square inch (psi) for an autoclave residence time of not less than 60 minutes; or
   ii. A temperature of not less than 135°C and a pressure of 31 psi for an autoclave residence time of not less than 45 minutes; or
   iii. A temperature of not less than 149°C and a pressure of 52 psi for an autoclave residence time of not less than 30 minutes.

II. When operating a vacuum autoclave, medical waste shall be subjected to a minimum of one prevacuum pulse to purge the autoclave of all air. The waste shall be subjected to the following:
   i. A temperature of not less than 121°C and pressure of 15 psi per an autoclave residence time of not less than 45 minutes; or
   ii. A temperature of not less than 135°C and a pressure of 31 psi for an autoclave residence time of not less than 30 minutes.

III. Medical waste shall not be considered properly treated unless the time, temperature and pressure indicators indicate mat the required time, temperature and pressure were reached during the autoclave process. If for any reasons, time temperature or pressure indicator indicates that the required temperature, pressure or residence time was not reached, the entire load of medical waste must be autoclaved again until the proper temperature, pressure and residence time were achieved.

IV. *Recording of operational parameters*: Each autoclave shall have graphic or computer recording devices which will automatically and continuously monitor and record dates, time of day, load identification number and operating parameters throughout the entire length of the autoclave cycle.

V. *Validation test spore testing*: The autoclave should completely and consistently kill approved biological indicator at the maximum design capacity of each autoclave unit. Biological indicator for autoclave shall be *Bacillus stearothermophilus* spores using vials or spore strips, with at least I × 10^4 spores per milliliter. Under no circumstances will an autoclave have minimum operating parameters less than a residence time of 30 minutes, regardless of temperature and pressure, a temperature less than 121°C or a pressure less than 15 psi.

VI. *Routine Test*: A chemical indicator strip/tape mat changes color when a certain temperature is reached can be used to verify that a specific temperature has been achieved. It may be necessary to use more than one strip one strip over the waste package at different location to ensure that the inner content of the package has been adequately autoclaved.

STANDARDS FOR LIQUID WASTE

The effluent generated from the hospital should conform to the following limits:

Parameters	**Permissible limits**
pH	6.5-9.0
Suspended solids	100 mg/L
Oil and grease	10 mg/L
BOD	30 mg/L
COD	250 mg/L
Bioassay test	90 percent survival of fish after 96 hours in 100 percent effluent

These limits are applicable to those hospitals which are either connected with sewers without terminal sewage treatment plant or not connected to public sewers. For discharge into public sewers with terminal facilities, the general standards as notified under the Environment (Protection) Act, 1986 shall be applicable.

STANDARDS OF MICROWAVING

1. Microwave treatment shall not be used for cytotoxic, hazardous or radioactive wastes, contaminated animal carcasses, body parts and large metal items.
2. The microwave system shall comply with the efficacy test/routine tests and a performance guarantee may be provided by the supplier before operation of the unit.
3. The microwave should completely and consistently kill the bacteria and other pathogenic organisms that is ensured by approved biological indicator at the maximum design capacity of each microwave unit. Biological indicators for microwave shall be *Bacillus subtilis* spores using vials or spore strips with at least 1×10^4 spores per milliliter.

STANDARDS FOR DEEP BURIAL

1. A pit or trench should be dug about 2 meters deep. It should be half filled with waste, then covered with lime within 50 cm of the surface, before filling the rest of the pit with soil.
2. It must be ensured that animals do not have any access to burial sites. Covers of galvanized iron/wire meshes may be used.
3. On each occasion, when wastes are added to the pit, a layer of 10 cm of soil shall be added to cover the wastes.
4. Burial must be performed under close and dedicated supervision.
5. The deep burial site should be relatively impermeable and no shallow well should be close to the site.
6. The pits should be distant from habitation, and sited so as to ensure that no contamination occurs of any surface water or groundwater. The area should not be prone to flooding or erosion.
7. The location of the deep burial site will be authorized by the prescribed authority.
8. The institution shall maintain a record of all pits for deep burial.

[1][SCHEDULE VI]

(See Rule 5)

SCHEDULE FOR WASTE MANAGEMENT FACILITIES LIKE INCINERATOR/ AUTOCLAVE/MICROWAVE SYSTEM

A. Hospitals and nursing homes in towns with population of 30 lakhs and above	By 30th June, 2000 or earlier
B. Hospitals and nursing homes in towns with population of below 30 lakhs:	
a. With 500 beds and above	By 30th June, 2000 or earlier
b. With 200 beds and above, but less than 500 beds	By 31st December, 2000 or earlier
c. With 50 beds and above, but less than 200 beds	By 31st December, 2001 or earlier
d. With less than 50 beds	By 31st December, 2002 or earlier
C. All other institutions generating bio-medical waste not included in A and B above.	By 31st December, 2002 or earlier.

[1]Substituted 'Schedule VI' by Rule 2 of the Biomedical Waste (M&H) (Amendment) Rules, 2000 notified vide notification SO 201(E), dated 6.3.2000 and came into force wef 6.3.2000.

FORM I

(See Rule 8)

[1]APPLICATION FOR AUTHORIZATION/RENEWAL OF AUTHORIZATION

(To be submitted in duplicate)

To,

The Prescribed Authority
(Name of the State Govt./UT Administration)
Address.

1. Particulars of Applicant
   i. Name of the Applicant
      (in block letters and in full)
   ii. Name of the Institution:
      Address:
      Tele No.
      Fax. No.
      Telex No.
2. Activity for which authorization is sought:
   i. Generation
   ii. Collection
   iii. Reception
   iv. Storage
   v. Transportation
   vi. Treatment
   vii. Disposal
   viii. Any other form of handling.
3. Please state whether applying for fresh authorization or for renewal: (in case of renewal previous authorization number and date)
4. i. Address of the institution handling biomedical wastes.
   ii. Address of the place of the treatment facility.
   iii. Address of the place of disposal of the waste.
5. i. Mode of transportation (in any) of biomedical waste.
   ii. Mode(s) of treatment.
6. Brief description of method of treatment and disposal (attach details):
7. i. Category (see Schedule I) of waste to be handled.
   ii. Quantity of waste (category-wise) to be handled per month.
8. **Declaration**

I do hereby declare that the statements made and information given above are true to the best of my knowledge and belief and that I have not concealed any information.

I do also hereby undertake to provide any further information sought by the prescribed authority in relation to these rules and to fulfill any conditions stipulated by the prescribed authority.

Date : Signature of the applicant

Place : Designation of the applicant

---

[1]Substituted by Rule 10 of the Biomedical Waste (M&H) (Second Amendment) Rules, 2000 notified vide SO 545(E), dated 2.6.2000.

FORM II

(See Rule 10)

ANNUAL REPORT

(To be submitted to the prescribed authority by 31st January every year).

1. Particulars of the applicant:
   i. Name of the authorized person(occupier/operator):
   ii. Name of the institution:
   Address
   Tel. No.
   Telex No.
   Fax No.
2. Categories of waste generated and quantity on a monthly average basis.
3. Brief details of the treatment facility.
   In case of off-site facility:
   i. Name of the operator
   ii. Name and address of the facility:
   Tel. No., Telex No., Fax No.
4. Category-wise quantity of waste treated.
5. Mode of treatment with details.
6. Any other information.
7. Certified that the above report is for the period from...................
   ....

Date : Signature ....

Place : Designation ....

FORM III
(See Rule 12)
ACCIDENT REPORTING

1. Date and time of accident.
2. Sequence of events leading to accident.
3. The waste involved in accident.
4. Assessment of the effects of the accidents on human health and the environment.
5. Emergency measures taken.
6. Steps taken to alleviate the effects of accidents.
7. Steps taken to prevent the recurrence of such an accident.

Date : Signature ....

Place : Designation ....

[1]FORM IV
[See Rule 8(4)]

(Authorization for operating a facility for collection, reception, treatment, storage, transport and disposal of biomedical wastes)

1. File number of authorization and date of issue...
2. ....of.. is hereby granted an authorization to operate a facility for collection, reception, storage, transport and disposal of biomedical waste on the premises situated at.
3. This authorization shall be in force for a period of...........................Years from the date of issue.
4. This authorization is subject to the conditions stated below and to such other conditions as may be specified in the rules for the time being in force under the Environment (Protection) Act, 1986.

Date : Signature ....

Place : Designation ....

Terms and conditions of authorization*

1. The authorization shall comply with the provisions of the Environment (Protection) Act, 1986 and the rules made thereunder.
2. The authorization or its renewal shall be produced for inspection at the request of an officer authorized by the prescribed authority.
3. The person authorized shall not rent, lend, sell, transfer or otherwise transport the biomedical wastes without obtaining prior permission of the prescribed authority.
4. Any unauthorized change in personnel, equipment or working conditions as mentioned in the application by the person authorized shall constitute a breach of his authorization.
5. It is the duty of the authorized person to take prior permission of the prescribed authority to close down the facility.

* Additional terms and conditions may be stipulated by the prescribed authority.

[1]Added by Rule 11 of the Biomedical Waste (M&H) (Second Amendment) Rules, 2000 notified vide SO 545(E), dated 2.6.2000.

[FORM V]
(See Rule 13)

Application for filing appeal against order passed by the prescribed authority at district level or regional office of the Pollution Control Board acting as prescribed authority or the State/Union Territory level authority.

1. Name and address of the person applying for appeal.
2. Number, date of order and address of the authority which passed the order, against which appeal is being made (certified copy of order to be attached).
3. Ground on which the appeal is being made.
4. List of enclosures other than the order referred in para 2 against which appeal is being filed.

Signature ....

Date : Name and address ....

F. No. 23(2)/96-HSMD
V. RAJAGOPALAN, Jt. Secretary

Note: The Principal rules were published in the Gazette of India vide number SO 630(E), dated 20.7.98 and subsequently amended vide (1) SO 201(E), dated 6.3.2000; (2) SO 545(E), dated 2.6.2000; and (111) SO1069(E), dated 17.9.2003.

Added by Rule 11 of the Biomedical Waste (M&H) (Second Amendment) Rules, 2000 notified vide SO 545 (E), dated 2.6.2000.

Abbreviations

AIDS	:	Acquired Immunodeficiency Syndrome
BMP	:	Best Management Practices
BMW	:	Biomedical Waste
CDC	:	Center for Disease Control
CWTF	:	Centralized Waste Treatment Facility
EtO	:	Ethylene Oxide
HBV	:	Hepatitis B Virus
HCF	:	Healthcare Faculty
HCV	:	Hepatitis C Virus
HCW	:	Healthcare Worker
HIV	:	Human Immunodeficiency Virus
ICO	:	Infection Control Officer
MoEF	:	Ministry of Environment and Forests
OSHA	:	Occupational Safety
PEP	:	Postexposure Prophylaxis
ppm	:	Parts per million
PVC	:	Polyvinyl Chloride
RVG	:	Radiovisiography
SEARO	:	Regional Office for South East Asia
UV	:	Ultraviolet
WHO	:	World Health Organization

References

1. A comprehensive immunization strategy to eliminate transmission of hepatitis B virus infection in the United States. Morbidity and Mortality weekly report 2006 Dec 8;55(RR-16).
2. Agarwal AG. Breaking the ice: a factsheet on exploring mercury and its alternatives. Hospital waste: Time to act: Srishti's factsheets on 14 priority areas; 2002 Jun.
3. Best management practices for amalgam waste. Illinois: American Dental Association; 2004.
4. Bhatti P. Sutlej mein fir mrit mili hazaron machhliyan. Dainik Bhaskar. 2009 Nov 19:1 (col. 2).
5. Biomedical waste management in Bangalore. Environmental Concerns [Online] [cited 2006 Jun 15]. Available from: URL:*http://kpspcb.kar.nic.in/ BMW/ environmental.htm.*
6. Biomedical waste management scenario in Delhi [Online] [cited 2010 Aug 16]. Available from: URL:*http://health.delhigovt.nic.in/Health/files/bio.html.*
7. Bulletin of Occupational and Environment Health. Workshop on Biomedical Waste Management-13.4.04. Ind Medica 2004;1(1):1-6.
8. Bulucea CAV, Bulucea AV, Popescu MC, Patrascu AF. Assessment of biomedical waste situation in hospitals of Dolj district. Int J Bio and Biomed Engg 2008;2(1):19-28.
9. CPR environmental education centre. Biomedical Waste Management. [Online]. [2005?] [cited 2010 Oct 14]. Available from: *URL:http://cpreec.org/ pubbook-biomedical.htm.*
10. C-Contents. [Online]. [cited 2010 Sept 28]; Available from: URL:*http://bmetpr.com/Hazardous%20Waste%20Management.pdf.*
11. CDC. 2009 H1N1 and seasonal flu: What you should know about flu antiviral drugs [Online] 2009 Oct 8 [cited 2010 Jul 7]. Available from: URL:*http://www.cdc.gov/H1N1flu/antivirals/geninfo.htm.*
12. CDC. 2009 H1N1 Influenza vaccine—inactivated (the "flu shot") what you need to know [Online] 2009 Oct 2 [cited 2010 Jul 7]. Available from: URL:*http://www.immunize.org/vis/h1n1_inactiveflu.pdf.*
13. CDC. 2009 H1N1("Swine Flu") and You [Online] 2010 Feb 10 [Cited 2010 Jul 7]. Available from: URL:*http://www.cdc.gov/h1n1flu/qa.htm.*

14. CDC. Information for pregnant women working in education, child care, and healthcare settings concerning 2009 H1N1 influenza virus. [Online]. 2009 Nov 9 [cited 2010 Jul 7]. Available from: URL:*http://www.cdc.gov/ h1n1flu/guidance/pregnant-hcw-educators.htm.*
15. CDC. Question and Answers: Antiviral drugs 2009-2010 flu season. [Online]. 2009 Nov 17 [cited 2010 Jul 7]. Available from: URL:*http://www.cdc.gov/ h1n1flu/antiviral.htm.*
16. CDC. Questions and answers: 2009 H1N1 nasal spray vaccine. [Online]. 2009 Oct 7 [cited 2010 Jul 7]. Available from: URL:*http://www.cdc.gov/ h1n1flu/ vaccination/nasalspray_qa.htm.*
17. CDC. Travelers' Health-Yellow Book. Atlanta: Mosby;2009.
18. CDC. Use of a reduced (4-dose) vaccine schedule for post exposure prophylaxis to prevent human rabies. Morbidity and Mortality weekly report 2010 Mar 19;59(02):1-9.
19. Centre for environment education and technology. Biomedical waste management – burgeoning issue [Online]. 2009 Aug 24 [cited 2010 Oct 14]; Available from: URL:*http://www.ceetindia.org/modules/news/article.php? storyid=40.*
20. Chandra H. Hospital waste—An environmental hazard and its management. Enviro News 1999 July; 5(3).
21. Chemical vapor sterilization. [Online]. [cited 2010 Oct 10]. Available from: URL:*http://www.tpub.com/content/medical/14274/css/14274_147.htm.*
22. Chitnis V, Vaidya K, Chitnis DS. Biomedical waste in laboratory medicine: Audit and management. Ind J Med Micro 2005;23(1):6-13.
23. Citizen consumer and Civic Action Group (CAG). Status report. Biomedical waste management practices in Chennai; September 2002.
24. Deliver, World Health Organization. Guidelines for the Storage of Essential Medicines and Other Health Commodities. Arlington: VA: John Snow, Inc.; 2003.
25. Dept. of Environment protection. Biomedical waste rule [Online] [cited 2010 Aug 27]; [12 screens]. Available from: URL:*http://www.fau.edu/ facilities/ehs/info/Biological-Waste-Program.pdf.*
26. Dogra TD, Rudra A. Lyon's Medical Jurisprudence and Toxicology. 11th edn. New Delhi: Delhi Law House; 2005.
27. Emmanuel J, Hrdinka C, Gruszyñski P, Waste Prevention Association Poland, Ralph Ryder, Communities Against Toxics UK, et al. Non-Incineration Medical Waste Treatment Technologies in Europe. Chlumova: Healthcare without Harm Europe; June 2004.

28. Environment Canada. Disposal of biomedical/pathological wastes. [Online]. 2005 Aug 15 [cited 2010 Aug 19]; Available from: URL:*http:// www.ec.gc.ca/ MERCURY/DA/ONBMP/EN/d_bio.cfm.*
29. Environmental health, safety, insurance and risk management. Biomedical waste management plan. University of North Florida; 2008 Jun.
30. ENVIS. Pondicherry Pollution Control Committee [Online]. 2006 July-Sept [cited 2010 Oct 11];[13 screens]. Available from: URL:*http:// dste.puducherry.gov.in/envisnew/FOURTH%20NEWSLETTER.pdf.*
31. Ethylene Oxide (EtO) sterilization process [Online] [cited 2010 Oct 14]. Available from: URL:*http://www.eurotherm-lifesciences.com/enGB/ applications/eto-sterilization/*
32. Ethylene oxide CAS no. 75-21-8. Report on carcinogens, eleventh edition [Online] [cited 2010 Apr 4]; [4 screens]. Available from: URL:*http://ntp.niehs.nih.gov/ntp/roc/eleventh/profiles/s085ethy.pdf.*
33. Farlex. The free dictionary [Online] [cited 2010 Sep 6]; Available from: URL:*http://encyclopedia.thefreedictionary.com/waste+minimization.*
34. Farlex. The free dictionary [Online] [cited 2010 Sep 6]; Available from: URL:*http://medical-dictionary.thefreedictionary.com/infection+ control.*
35. FLU.GOV.Vaccination [Online]. 2010 Apr 25 [cited 2010 Aug 26]. Available from: URL:*http://www.flu.gov/individualfamily/vaccination/ index.html.*
36. Frequently asked question about 2009 H1N1 Live attenuated intranasal vaccine (H1N1 nasal spray vaccine) [Online] [cited 2010 Apr 25]. Available from: URL:*http://www.sccvote.org/SCC/docs/ Public%20Health %20Department%20(DEP)/attachments/FAQ_H1N1_ Nasal_Spray_FAQs.pdf.*
37. Gabela SD. Healthcare Waste Management in Public Clinics in the Ilembe District: A Situational Analysis. Durban: Health Systems Trust; 2007.
38. Guidelines for management of biomedical waste in the Northwest Territories. 2005 April. [Online] [cited 2010 Aug 18]. Available from: URL:*http://www.enr.gov.nt.ca/_live/documents/documentManager Upload/biomedical_waste.pdf.*
39. Gujarat Pollution Control Board. Towards a healthy future: Biomedical waste management. [Online] [cited 2010 Oct 14];[35 screens]. Available from: URL:*http://gpcb.gov.in/bmw_ws.pdf.*
40. Hegde V, Kulkarni RD, Ajantha GS. Biomedical waste management. J Oral and Max Path 2007;11(1):5-9.

41. Human rabies prevention –United States. Morbidity and Mortality weekly report 1999 Jan 08;48(RR-1):1-21.
42. Hydroclave system corp. Medical waste solutions [Online] [cited 2010 Aug 17]. Available from: URL:*http://www.hydroclave.com/tech_detail.html.*
43. Hydroclave: An ecofriendly solution for biomedical waste mgmt. Hospi Medica India 2002. [Online] [cited 2010 Apr 4]. Available from: URL:*http://www.expresshealthcaremgmt. com/20020228/medica14.shtml.*
44. Joshi S, Walawalkar V, Hajirnis V, Date P, Kadam R. Managing municipal solid waste: special focus on biomedical waste management—a case study. [Online] [cited 2010 Oct 18]; [10 screens]. Available from: URL: *http://wgbis.ces.iisc.ernet.in/energy/lake2006/programme/programme/lake2006_Pdf/Sanjay_Joshi.pdf.*
45. Kishore J, Goel P, Sagar B, Joshi TK. Awareness about biomedical waste management and infection control among dentists of a teaching hospital in New Delhi, India. Indian J Dent Res 2000 Oct-Dec; 11(4):157-61.
46. Kishore J, Ingle GK. Biomedical waste management in India. New Delhi: Century Publications; 2004.
47. Madhya Pradesh Pollution Control Board. Handling of biomedical waste. [Online] [cited 2010 Oct 14]. Available from: URL:*http://www.mppcb.nic.in/Bio_Categories.htm#Top.*
48. Manyele SV. Effects of improper hospital waste management on occupational health and safety. Afr Newslett on Occup Health and Safety 2004;14:30-33.
49. MedImmune, LLC. 100126_clean Influenza A (H1N1) 2009 Monovalent Vaccine Live, Intranasal_USPI_submitted [ID09H0101]+ WHO. US Government License No. 1799. [Online] [cited 2010 Aug 26]; [22 screens]. Available from: URL:*http://www.fda.gov/downloads/BiologicsBlood Vaccines/Approved Products/UCM182406.pdf.*
50. Miller GA. The H1N1 swine flu vaccine is here: Should you get it? Updated October 1st [Online]. 2009 Sep 18 [cited 2010 Apr 24]. Available from: URL:*http://thefastertimes.com/clinicalupdate/2009/09/18/faqs-about-the-h1n1-vaccine/*
51. Ministry of Environment and Forests, Notification. The biomedical waste (Management and Handling) rules, 1998. [Online]. 1998 Jul 20 [cited 2010 Oct 14]; [27 screens]. Available from URL:*http://www.ppcb.gov. in/BMW/BMW%20Rule.pdf.*

52. Ministry of Environment and Forests. Notification. New Delhi; 1998 July 20.
53. Ministry of Health and Family Welfare, Government of India. Infection Management and Environment Plan. Policy framework. March 2007.
54. Ministry of Health, Ministry of Environment, Ministry of Advanced Education, Employment and Labour. Saskatchewan biomedical waste management guidelines. Feb 2008. Available from: *URL:http://www.health.gov.sk.ca/biomedical-waste-management.*
55. Ministry of public health, Afghanistan. Infection management and environment plan. Islamic Republic of Afghanistan; 2009 Aug 11.
56. Pandit NA, Tabish SA, Qadri GJ, Mustafa A. Biomedical waste management in a large teaching hospital. Hospital Today 2007 Jan-March;14(1):57-59.
57. National guidelines on hospital waste management based upon the biomedical waste (Management and Handling) rules, 1998. [Online] [cited 2010 Mar 23];[6 screens]. Available from: URL:*http://www.maha-arogya.gov.in/ actsrules/Biomedical/Biomedical.pdf.*
58. Nazareth S, Rathi MK. Harbouring an unnecessary evil: A factsheet on mercury in health set ups. Hospital waste: Time to act: Srishti's factsheets on 14 priority areas. 2002 Jun.
59. Nema SK, Ganeshprasad. Plasma pyrolysis of medical waste. Current Science 2002 Aug 10; 83(3):271-8.
60. New Hampshire department of environmental services pollution prevention program and the New Hampshire dental society. Best management practices for dental offices in New Hampshire; 2002 Jan.
61. Northeast Natural Resource Centre of the National Wildlife Federation and The Vermont State Dental Society. The Environmentally Responsible Dental Office: A Guide to Proper Waste Management in Dental Offices; Jun 1999.
62. Office of Risk Management (ORM). Biomedical waste disposal procedures. University of Ottawa. [Online] [2007] [cited 2010 Oct 14]. Available from: URL:*http://www.uottawa.ca/services/ehss/docs/BiomedicalWasteDisposal ProceduresSept07.pdf.*
63. Patil AD, Shekdar AV. Healthcare waste management in India. J Enviro Manag 2001 Oct;63(2):211-20.
64. Persistent Organic Pollutants: A global issue, a global response. [Online]. [cited 2010 Apr 15]. Available from: URL:*http://www.epa.gov/ international/toxics/pop.htm.*

65. Prevention of hepatitis A through active or passive immunization. Morbidity and Mortality weekly report 2006 May 19; 55(RR-7).
66. Pruss A, Giroult E, Rushbrook P, editors. Safe management of wastes from healthcare activities. Geneva: World Health Organization; 1999.
67. Pruss A, Townsend WK. Teacher's Guide. Management of wastes from healthcare activities. Geneva: World Health Organization; 1998.
68. Punjab State Council for science and technology. Environmental Information system. Biomedical waste [Online]. [cited 2010 Oct 14]; Available from: URL:*http://www.punjabenvironment.com/swmgmt_BMW.htm.*
69. Qureshi W, Hassan G, Wani NA, Baba A, Kadri SM, Khan N. Awareness of biomedical waste management amongst staff of the government SMHS hospital, Srinagar—A tertiary level hospital in the Kashmir valley. Hospital's Today 2007;14(1):60-1.
70. Radha KV, Kalaivani K, Lavanya R. A case study of biomedical waste management in hospitals. Glob J Health Sci 2009 Apr;1(1):82-8.
71. Rasmussen CD, Rasmussen, Rasmussen and Charowsky. Treatment of biomedical waste with ozone [Online]. [2007?] [cited 2010 Oct 14]; [12 screens]. Available from: URL: *http://www.envirosolutions.net/Treatment_ of_Biomedical_Waste_with_Ozone.pdf.*
72. Rau EH, Alaimo RJ, Ashbrook PC, Austin SM, Borenstein N, Evans MR, et al. Minimization and management of wastes from Biomedical Research. Env Health Pers 2000 Dec;108 Suppl 6: 955.
73. Recommended adult immunization schedule, United States, Oct 2005-Sept 2006. Morbidity and Mortality weekly report 2005 Oct 14;54(40).
74. Roberson TM, Heymann HO, Swift EJ, editors. Art and Science of Operative Dentistry. 4th edn. Missouri: Mosby; 2002.
75. Rutala WA, Weber DJ, Healthcare Infection Control Practices Advisory Committee (HICPAC). Guideline for disinfection and sterilization in healthcare facilities, 2008.
76. Safety services office. Autoclave Safety—Guidance for university departments and functions. Leicester: University of Leicester; 2000.
77. Sarojini E, Jayanthi S, Venkatraman JS, Prashanthini K. Performance study on common biomedical waste treatment facility, Chettipalayam, Coimbatore. Proceedings of the International conference on Sustainable Solid Waste Management; 2007 Sept 5-7; Chennai, India. 182-88.
78. Secretariat of the Basel Convention. Technical guidelines on the environmentally sound management on biomedical and healthcare wastes (Y1;Y3) Sept 2003.

79. Sheth KN, Desai PH. Characterization and management of biomedical waste in SAE hospital, Anand—A case study. EJEAFChe ISSN:1579-4377 2006;5(6):1583-9.
80. Sikri VK. Fundamentals of dental radiology. 4th edn. New Delhi: CBS; 2010.
81. Singh R. Impact of needlestick injuries on healthcare workers. Srishti Toxic Lin 2004 Mar;20:1-4.
82. Singh R. Waste management: A timely prescription. Toxic Lin 2004 Dec;24:1-4.
83. Singh VP, Biswas G, Sharma JJ. Biomedical waste management—An emerging concern in Indian hospitals. Ind J Foren Med Toxic 2007;1(1);7-12.
84. Singh Z, Bhalwar R, Jayaram J, Tilak VW. An introduction to essentials of Biomedical waste management. MJAFI;57:144-7.
85. Snelling G. Autoclave validation—What is really required? [Online]. [cited 2010 Aug 19]; [4 screens]. Available from: URL:*http://www.intercal.co.za/ pdf/acvalid.pdf*
86. Suite101®.com. Sanofi Pasteur, Inc. H1N1 vaccine ingredients—swine flu injection package insert contents and dosage information. [Online]. 2009 Nov 4 [cited 2010 Aug 26]. Available from: URL:*http://public-healthcare-issues.suite101.com/article.cfm/sanofi_pasteur_inc_h1n1_vaccine_ingredients.*
87. Swinwood JF, Waite TD, Kruger P, Rao SM. Radiation technologies for waste treatment: A global perspective. IAEA Bulletin 1/1994.
88. Tandon A. Cobalt-60 imported as industrial waste? The Tribune. 2010 Apr 12:1 (col. 5).
89. The environmentally responsible dental office: A guide to proper waste management in Connecticut dental office. Northeast natural resource center of the national wildlife federation and state of Connecticut, department of environmental protection; 2000 June.
90. US Food and Drug Administration. Influenza (H1N1) 2009 Monovalent vaccines-descriptions and ingredients. [Online]. 2009 Nov 16 [cited 2010 Aug 26]. Available from: URL:*http://www.fda.gov/BiologicsBlood Vaccines/Vaccines/QuestionsaboutVaccines/ucm186102.htm.*
91. United Nations Environment Programme/SBC. Preparation of national healthcare waste management plans in Subsaharan countries. Guidance manual. Secretariat of Basel Convention and World Health Organization; [2005?]
92. Updated US public health service guidelines for the management of occupational exposures to HIV and recommendations for postexposure

prophylaxis. Morbidity and Mortality weekly report 2005 Sep 30;54(RR-9).

93. Updated US public health service guidelines for the management of occupational exposures to HBV, HCV, and HIV and recommendations for postexposure prophylaxis. Morbidity and Mortality weekly report 2001 Jun 29;50(RR-11).
94. Virginia Dental Association, Virginia department of environmental quality. The Environmentally –Responsible dental office: A guide to pollution prevention and proper waste management in dental offices. Richmond: Virginia Dental Association; 2005.
95. West Bengal Pollution Control Board. Health care waste management scenario in West Bengal. [Online]. [2009?] [cited 2010 Oct 14];[14 screens]. Available from: URL: *http://www. wbpcb.gov.in/html/downloads/bmw report.pdf.*
96. Worker Health Chartbook 2004. NIOSH Publication no. 2004-146 [Online]. [cited 2010 Jul 7]. Available from: URL: *http://www.cdc.gov/niosh/docs/ 2004-146/ch2/ch2-10.asp.htm.*
97. Workshop on biomedical waste management in Indian hospitals: trends, technology and challenge. [Online]. 2009 May 27 [cited 2010 Mar 27). Available from: URL: *http://www. clickindia.com/detail.php?id=1436719.*
98. World Health Organization. Practical guidelines for infection control in healthcare facilities. SEARO Regional Publication No. 41. New Delhi: WPRO Regional Publication; 2004.
99. World Health Organization. Safe healthcare waste management. Policy paper.[Online]. 2004 Aug [cited 2010 Aug 19]; [2 screens]. Available from: URL:*http://www.who.int/immunization_safety/publications/waste_management/en/safe_health_care_waste_management_ policy.pdf.*
100. World Health Organization. Safe management of biomedical sharps waste in India—A report on alternative treatment and nonburn disposal practices. New Delhi: WHO regional office for South-East Asia; 2005.
101. Yadav M. Hospital waste – A major problem. JK- Practi 2001;8(4):276-82.

Index

Page numbers followed by *f* refer to figures and *t* refer to tables